NUTRITION AND DIET RESEARCH PROGRESS

GREEN TEA AND BEYOND

NUTRITION AND DIET RESEARCH PROCESSES

Additional books in this series can be found on Nova's website under the Series tab.

Additional E-books in this series can be found on Nova's website under the E-books tab.

NUTRITION AND DIET RESEARCH PROGRESS

GREEN TEA AND BEYOND

STEPHEN HSU
WITH
CHRISTINE HURLEY DERISO

Nova Biomedical
Nova Science Publishers, Inc.
New York

For permission to use material from this book please contact us:
Telephone 631-231-7269; Fax 631-231-8175
Web Site: http://www.novapublishers.com

LIBRARY OF CONGRESS CATALOGING-IN-PUBLICATION DATA
Deriso, Christine Hurley, 1961-
Green tea and beyond / Christine Hurley Deriso and Stephen Hsu.
p. ; cm.
Includes bibliographical references and index.
ISBN 978-1-61668-845-5 (softcover)
1. Green tea--Health aspects. 2. Green tea--Therapeutic use. I. Hsu, Stephen. II. Title.
[DNLM: 1. Tea. 2. Phytotherapy. WB 438 D795g 2010]
RM251.D47 2010
615'.321--dc22-2010015589

Published by Nova Science Publishers, Inc. ✢ New York

CONTENTS

PREFACE

This book discusses the values of Green Tea as having anti-oxidant benefits as well as healing attributes. When I moved from China to the United States as a young man, I was struck by an observation that was too obvious to ignore. Green tea consuming Asians, in many ways, are healthier than Americans. They have less cancer of the mouth, colon, prostate and bladder; less cardiovascular disease; and less obesity and high blood pressure. They have less disfiguring rheumatoid arthritis, lupus and other autoimmune diseases in which the body inexplicably attacks its own tissues. They even have fewer wrinkles. Some diseases are virtually nonexistent in China and Japan, such as xerostamia, or dry mouth, which affects fully a third of elderly Americans.

Let's narrow the lens and zoom in just on Japan, where humans enjoy the longest lifespan of any country in the world. The Japanese life expectancy of 82.2 years contrasts with an American life expectancy of 77.2 years. Japan has almost no natural resources, the workforce is under tremendous stress, the suicide rate is almost three times higher than in the United States and the Japanese consume more cigarettes per person. Yet on average, they still live five years longer than Americans. What gives?

Chapter I - I can wax poetic for hours about the healing properties of green tea—and I find more of those properties every day in my Medical College of Georgia laboratory—but I always temper my enthusiasm with a sobering, if clichéd, reality: There's no magic pill, or tea leaf, for that matter, that will cure all ills. Life just is not that simple. Our bodies are far too complex—marvelously, amazingly so—to respond to a one size fits all approach to wellness.

Chapter II - My adopted state of Georgia does not have an official beverage, but if it did, there is no doubt what it would be: sweet tea, loaded with sugar.

America was slower than Asia to warm to the charms of tea, but once iced tea was introduced at the World's Fair in St. Louis in 1904, the country—particularly the South—was hooked. When tea bags hit the scene four years later, Americans never looked back.

Chapter III - When a colleague of mine at the Medical College of Georgia recently diagnosed a patient with a cancerous tongue lesion, she scheduled surgery to remove the lesion. Of course, this meant the patient would lose part of her tongue—a sad and often debilitating consequence of oral cancer.

The alternative—unchecked cancer growth—obviously was unthinkable, and the patient resigned herself to her fate. She agreed to return for surgery several weeks later.

Chapter IV - Let us imagine for a moment that you are holding a bruised apple. Those spongy brown spots make the apple pretty unappetizing. But before you take a bite, someone offers you a potion that can be applied to the brown spots, making the apple look shiny and lustrous. Now, mind you, the brown spots have not gone away. They just look better. But the apple is still damaged.

Chapter V - I am a basic scientist, as opposed to a clinical scientist, which means my research takes place in a lab. I have wonderful colleagues who can take my results to the next step by testing them on patients, but early in the process, my work is a solitary affair.

Chapter VI - You can tell a lot about a culture from its advertisements.

In my native country, China, most television commercials are about skin care products and medications. In my adopted country, the United States, most are about food, drinks and cars. My tongue-in-cheek theory is that manufacturers want us to eat until we are so fat that we cannot walk anymore … at which point it is time to buy a car. (Okay, maybe it is not so tongue-in-cheek.)

Chapter VII - Remember the skin conditions, such as dandruff and psoriasis, that I referenced in Chapter Five? Many of them belong to a big disease group: autoimmune diseases, the third largest category of diseases in the country, after heart diseases and cancer. There are more than sixty-five types affecting eight percent of the U.S. population—a whopping 25 million people. Each year, we spend approximately $120 billion treating these diseases.

Chapter VIII - I suspected a link between green tea consumption and Sjogren's syndrome because EGCG, that powerhouse of polyphenols, is known to suppress inflammation. Inflammation results when the immune system mounts a defense to a real or perceived enemy. Since EGCG suppresses inflammation, it should affect the magnitude of an autoimmune response.

Chapter IX - I spent a considerable amount of time in Chapters Seven and Eight discussing dry mouth, or xerostomia.

If this problem—the inability to form sufficient saliva—strikes you as a mild inconvenience, or perhaps vaguely unfortunate, I guarantee that you have been fortunate enough not to experience it.

Chapter X - The information presented in this book thus far is, admittedly, a lot to swallow.

Can the leaves from a simple plant that grows in abundance really help treat cancer, obesity, skin conditions and autoimmune diseases, among other conditions?

Chapter XI - As I have walked you through the health benefits of green tea in the preceding chapters of this book, I am mindful that skepticism may persist.

Maybe you are thinking: *This is all too good to be true.* Heaven knows we are inundated with enough spurious health claims to wonder if each new 'guaranteed product' is nothing more than snake oil.

Chapter XII - First, I need to say that there is no miracle drug, or miracle drink, or miracle green tea. There are a lot of scientifically validated benefits of green tea, including those generated by some of the best medical centers in the United States, such as the Mayo Clinic and MD Anderson Cancer Center. We now even have a "green tea drug" – Veregen, approved by the Food and Drug Administration.

About the Authors

Dr. Stephen Hsu, Associate Professor at the Medical College of Georgia, earned a Bachelor's Degree in Biochemistry from Wuhan University in China, a Master's Degree in Molecular Biology from Montclair State University in New Jersey and a Ph.D. in Cell Biology and Anatomy from the University of Cincinnati, College of Medicine. He completed a Postdoctoral Fellowship at Memorial Sloan-Kettering Cancer Center in New York City. After four years as a television commentator and host for ESPN International, Dr. Hsu taught at the National University of Singapore prior to receiving the Ruth L. Kirstein Research Service Award from the National Cancer Institute, and conducted cancer research at New York University. He is a past president of the Georgia Chapter of the American Association for Dental Research and a member of the American Association for Cancer Research and the International Association for Dental Research. He has authored more than forty articles in peer-reviewed scientific journals and has presented his research findings at scientific meetings worldwide. He has consistently served as reviewer of grant applications for the National Institutes of Health, US Department of Defense, and the National University of Singapore and for more than twelve scientific journals. Dr. Hsu's research has been funded by the National Institutes of Health and the U.S. Department of Defense, among other organizations. Dr. Hsu has collaborated with researchers representing the fields of oral biology/maxillofacial pathology, dermatology, molecular biology and oral surgery at Columbia University, Baylor College of Medicine and research institutions in China, India and Japan, among other institutions. He partnered with fitness expert Denise Austin and CCA Industries Inc. to develop everyday skin care products, and many other green tea-containing consumer products such as Mega-T green tea chewing gum and mints, Sudden Change and

ScarZone skin care products, and Nutra Nail products, that deliver the healing properties of green tea and has patented additional related innovations. Dr. Hsu filed two patents in 2005 on autoimmune diseases and formulations for consumer products, and two additional patents in 2009 on flu prevention and dry mouth management. In 2005, Dr. Hsu received the Creativity Award from the Medical College of Georgia. He is included in *Who's Who in America* and *Who's Who in American Education* for the 60th diamond edition of 2006. He and wife Tracy live in Augusta, Georgia with their sons, Alexander and Andrew.

Christine Hurley Deriso earned a Bachelor's Degree in Journalism and has served as the Publications Editor at the Medical College of Georgia for more then twenty years. Her first book, *Dreams to Grow On,* was published by Illumination Arts in 2002 and was named an Outstanding Book of the Year by the Independent Publishers Association. She has published three novels with Random House. She has written feature articles and humor essays for national magazines including *Ladies' Home Journal, Parents, Family Circle* and *Child.* She lives in North Augusta, South Carolina with her husband, Graham, and their children, Gregory and Julianne. Green tea has been a regular part of her diet since she began working with Dr. Hsu in 2001.

ACKNOWLEDGMENTS

I always consider my self lucky to work with people rich in knowledge and diverse in expertise. Particularly in this information era, individualism has a small chance for success, simply because one cannot process the voluminous information available without collaboration.

All of my success reflects collaboration, and I am eternally grateful for those who have helped smooth my path and advance my journey.

First, I would like to thank my childhood peers. My early experiences in table tennis and basketball honed my appreciation for teamwork. That lesson was reinforced tenfold when the idyllic stage of my childhood was brutally and abruptly replaced with my involuntary service on the 53rd Farm during China's Cultural Revolution. I will always honor and cherish the unfortunate boys and girls who worked by my side. We are survivors, and proud of it.

Once I was allowed to resume my education as a young man, I discovered a wellspring of likeminded individuals at Wuhan University, where most of us believe that we spent the best time of our life for our careers, our dreams and our future. (We are planning a 30-year reunion in 2012.)

I also thank my colleagues at ESPN, where I worked as a sports anchor for four years. Everyone, from producers to production assistants, pulled together and afforded me the pleasure and privilege of broadcasting sports on live television.

My dedication to teamwork has grown even stronger during my research career. My work would not be possible without the contributions of many fine scientists, both at the Medical College of Georgia and beyond, including Drs. Xian Qiang Yang, C.S. Yang, Hasan Mukhtar, Ping Chen, Yukihiko Hara, Douglas Dickinson, Nihal Ahmed, Santosh Katiyar, Tetsuya Yamamoto, Tokio Osaki, Isamu Kodani, Carol Lapp, Scott DeRossi, Kalu Ogbureke,

George Schuster, Douglas Walsh, Wendy Bollag, Jill Lewis, John Wataha, Kevin Gillespie, Jaime Hughes, Haiyan Qin, Yat-Ho Ma, among many others.

I am also grateful to Dr. Connie Drisko, Dean of School of Dentistry, for her strong support for my research on green tea, and my students at the Medical College of Georgia, many of whom have helped advance my research. (Their skills at table tennis are more debatable; I challenge every freshman class to beat me at the game, promising A's in biochemistry if they succeed. No one has handed me a defeat yet, though plenty have earned their A's honestly!)

My research has opened exciting doors to entrepreneurialism, and I am deeply indebted to people who helped make that happen, including CCA Industries CEO and Founder David Edell. (A quick aside: During my initial meeting with David, he said, "Steve, the data you presented to us are very convincing, but all this information has been published and is in the public domain; so what do we need you for?" My answer was simple: "Well, you don't! But without me, your products will be no different than the ones you're competing against." It seems my answer wasn't bad: we have been working together since 2004.)

A very special person for me to thank is my partner for writing this book: Christine Deriso. We have worked on this project for three years now. It would be impossible to complete this book without her hard work.

Of course, my biggest debt of gratitude goes to my family. I am so lucky to have a wonderful wife, Tracy, and our A Team, sons Alex and Andrew. (The A Team isn't a reference to the television show, but to my expectations about grades!) My wife was a successful television anchor and model when love at first sight struck us at a social event at the Memorial Sloan-Kettering Cancer Center. She has encouraged and supported me every step of the way, including by urging me to ditch junk food and cigarettes early in our relationship. She also sacrificed her career for my own, selling a successful business to be a full time mom when our sons came on the scene. There is no way that I could achieve any thing without her love and support.

INTRODUCTION

Green tea hasn't always been a source of intrigue for me. For years, it was a source of misery.

I was eleven years old when my idyllic childhood in Beijing, China came to a brutal and abrupt end. I was born to wealth and privilege as a descendant of Shi-Chang Hsu (pronounced "shu"), president of the Republic of China from 1918 to 1922. My sister and I were raised in a home with maids, chefs, a chauffer … even a "milk mother*"

My father was an economist, my mother an architect. My sister and I were eager to do well in school and follow in our family's high achieving footsteps.

Fate intervened in the form of a political and social storm that turned China upside down. China's Cultural Revolution, a ten-year experiment in creating an egalitarian society by uplifting the poor and stripping the affluent of their wealth, began in 1966 and ended life as it was known for millions of Chinese – my family included.

A DESCENT INTO HELL: MY LIFE AS A 'LITTLE DOG'

Mao Zedong, the infamous leader of the Cultural Revolution, envisioned Maoism (or called "Mao Zedong Thoughts)—a mangled hybrid of socialism and Chinese imperialism that was mostly an exercise in unbridled power and egoism run amok—as a great leveling device. Toward that end, he

* A woman who is paid to breastfeed an unrelated child.

systematically purged the country of intellectuals, often through humiliation, torture and imprisonment.

That being the case, our family was probably fortunate, because my parents' lives were spared. But I didn't feel fortunate. My family was forced to surrender every asset to the government. We were expelled from the capital city, Beijing, to the central city of Wuhan. My New York University educated father was ordered to perform menial labor in a factory, earning a meager salary and living apart from my mother, sister and me. He was granted one day visits biweekly.

My sister, mother and I were moved into a one-room hovel and relied on subsistence level rations of food and everything from coal to matches. Adding to our anguish was the fact that we were now stigmatized. We were called capitalist puppies—little dogs. In China, "dog" is the ultimate denigration.

I was appalled at the injustice and contemplated trying to escape the country. But what could I do? Where could I go? I was only a child, and even my parents seemed powerless to relieve our growing desperation.

What should have been my one source of hope—the news that my sister and I would be allowed to continue our schooling—proved to be nothing more than a cruel joke. The school was managed by uneducated peasants and soldiers who taught nothing but loyalty to Chairman Mao and the regime. We learned nothing, not even the alphabet. We just played sports and fought with each other.

I couldn't imagine that life could get worse—yet it did. After completing ninth grade, I was told that my "education" was over.

Cold Mountain

I was wrenched from my home at the age of 16 and trucked to a labor camp called the 53rd Farm, housed on an isolated mountain. Working alongside other boys and girls, many of whom shared my crime of being born to educated parents, we were forced to farm the land and create our own food and lodging. Before we built shelter, we had to live in a mud-made structure that housed water buffaloes. We cleaned out the manure to make space to sleep. There was no electricity, no heat, no running water, no sewage system … no nothing. What we had in abundance were fleas, mosquitoes, leeches, flies, maggots and countless other parasites.

We worked eighteen hour days, building a dam, raising pigs and growing rice, vegetables and tea leaves. I vividly remember standing waist-deep in a rice paddy with sweat pouring from my brow and leeches digging into my flesh. Fleas and mosquitoes feasted on our skin as we slept. We drank water from the same pond where water buffaloes and pigs bathed, so diarrhea was constant. I have intestinal problems to this day. Injuries also were common. I remember breaking my leg with a dirt cart.

But no matter how ill or injured we were, work was mandatory. Our survival depended on our salary—about sixty-seven cents a day—and malingerers were severely punished. Our only break was an annual visit home during Chinese New Year.

Once we harvested our first crop of tea leaves, green tea replaced water as our source of fluid. As I thirstily drank the beverage that was provided during breaks in the field, I had no idea that I had unwittingly tapped into one of nature's most healthful resources. That knowledge would come later … much later.

At that point, my sole preoccupation was survival.

A Death Grip on Hope

Hope was all I had left. Like a toddler clutching a favorite blanket, I kept a death grip on happy memories of my big family, comfortable home and unlimited potential. It all seemed like a dream now, but I could not shake the sense that joy was somehow within reach, if I could just keep putting one foot in front of the other.

Then one day, something extraordinary happened. Like the sun peeking through the clouds after a violent storm, my chance materialized. In 1976, the Cultural Revolution sputtered to its demise. As abruptly as it had begun, it was over. I was transferred to a small farm near Wuhan, where my family still lived. No more labor camps. No more persecution. No more sleeping with water buffaloes or sharing the same filthy water.

My top priority was to resume my education. My family provided resources to buy chemistry, physics, math and English books so I could study for the college entrance examination. Farm work still dominated my days, but in the evenings when my coworkers played poker or watched movies, I was hitting the books, interspersing studies with calisthenics to stay warm in my unheated quarters. (I was relatively free, but still poor.)

Despite my dedication, I lost so much ground over the years that the effort sometimes seemed futile. I knew nothing about math or science. Chemistry was as foreign as an unfamiliar language. But I remembered how to read and write. That was my springboard. If I could read, I could learn. And I had no higher priority. I never felt so driven in my life. My chance, miraculously, had materialized, and I was not about to blow it.

A New Beginning

A year after my release from the 53rd Farm, I felt I had learned enough to take a college entrance exam. So I took it … and failed. I was 22.

But the setback only made me redouble my efforts. I went back to my hometown of Tianjin, about a hundred miles from Beijing, stayed in my aunt's house and studied twenty hours a day, supplementing my efforts with help from tutors. I had to pass that college entrance exam if I had any hope for a satisfying future.

Three months later, I took the test again—and passed with flying colors. I was suddenly welcomed at the Chinese university of my choice. I immediately enrolled in Wuhan University (which as of 2005 produced more U.S. professors than any other Chinese university). Finally, I reached the destination I envisioned as a young child—a place a world apart from the mountain where I grew tea trees.

I earned a degree in biochemistry, then came to the United States for graduate work. I did not speak English, but my enthusiasm was so boundless that I barely recognized that as a limitation. I studied English as a second language in Le Mars, Iowa, then with the help of my uncle Henry, I took the Graduate Record Examination and enrolled at Montclair State University in New Jersey, where I earned a Master of Arts degree and worked two jobs to support myself. By the time I enrolled in the University of Cincinnati School of Medicine in 1985, my academic record was rewarded with a scholarship. I earned a Ph.D. in cell biology and anatomy in 1991.

Coming Full Circle

Today, my life has come full circle. Instead of growing tea trees in a labor camp, I am working in a laboratory studying their amazing healing properties.

The symbolism is not lost on me. In the midst of my despair on that wretched mountain, I was surrounded by a wellspring of hope and vitality, growth and abundance. I was immersed in the plant that I would come to find more fascinating than any other on earth.

I have devoted my career to learning more about green tea, and I never lose sight of the impetus for my curiosity. As I peer into microscopes and study cultures in my Medical College of Georgia laboratory, I think of the youths who never made it off the mountain. Sometimes, the memories are overwhelming. But more often than not, those memories propel me forward. Hope springs eternal, even on an isolated mountain farmed by sad, lost children. I dedicate my research to those lost children, and to the hope for an ever improving world. The resources, I have learned, are right at our fingertips.

Chapter I

It's Written in the Tea Leaves

A Tale of Two Countries: Why the Health Disparity?

I can wax poetic for hours about the healing properties of green tea—and I find more of those properties every day in my Medical College of Georgia laboratory—but I always temper my enthusiasm with a sobering, if clichéd, reality: There's no magic pill, or tea leaf, for that matter, that will cure all ills. Life just is not that simple. Our bodies are far too complex—marvelously, amazingly so—to respond to a one size fits all approach to wellness.

But when I moved from China to the United States as a young man, I was struck by an observation that was too obvious to ignore. Green tea consuming Asians, in many ways, are healthier than Americans.

They just are.

They have less cancer of the mouth, colon, prostate and bladder; less cardiovascular disease; and less obesity and high blood pressure. They have less disfiguring rheumatoid arthritis, lupus and other autoimmune diseases in which the body inexplicably attacks its own tissues. They even have fewer wrinkles.

Some diseases are virtually nonexistent in China and Japan, such as xerostamia, or dry mouth, which affects fully a third of elderly Americans.

Let's narrow the lens and zoom in just on Japan, where humans enjoy the longest lifespan of any country in the world. The Japanese life expectancy of 82.2 years contrasts with an American life expectancy of 77.2 years. Japan has almost no natural resources, the workforce is under tremendous stress, the suicide rate is almost three times higher than in the United States and the Japanese consume more cigarettes per person. Yet on average, they still live five years longer than Americans.

What Gives?

Certainly, Asian and American cultures are different in so many ways that several things could conceivably account for these generalities (and that is just what they are—generalities). But no one can deny the growing evidence that our health is greatly influenced by how we fuel our bodies. We have always known this on some level, even intuitively. Some foods make us feel energetic, others sluggish. Some cause constipation, others help keep us regular. Some contribute to obesity, others to a healthy weight. So no one will find it earth shattering that one of nature's drinks—tea—affects the functioning of the human body, just as a high octane fuel affects the functioning of a car.

Building on the Wisdom of Our Ancestors

Although I have delved into the subject in a highly scientific way, people throughout millennia have intuited and anecdotally demonstrated the healing properties of green tea.

Green tea is an integral part of the Asian culture. Fully 98 percent of Japanese adults drink it regularly, as do a large percentage of Chinese. Why? Because they have learned from centuries of folklore, anecdotal evidence and conventional wisdom that the beverage is good for them.

Folklore about tea abounds in Asia, as in much of the world. The earliest Chinese literature indicates that the Chinese grew and used tea plants 3,000 years ago. In 2737 B.C., Chinese Emperor Shen-Nung placed camellia blossom tips into a cup of boiled water and pronounced the beverage healing and refreshing.

Tea consumption began in earnest around 200 B.C., popularized when it was said to cure the ailing troops of General Zhu Ge Liang (Kong Ming). During the Tang Dynasty (618-907), tea became an essential component of Chinese culture. Chinese author Lu Yu (733-804) at age twenty-eight published the book, *Cha Jing* (literally, The Book of Tea), systematically chronicling the planting, processing, preparation and consumption of tea. If you want to learn all the history of tea, the best place to go is the Tea Museum in Hangzhou, China.

Japan was the first country to import tea and tea culture from China, probably during the Tang Dynasty when the countries exchanged priests. Japan's "tea culture," which incorporated cultural, spiritual and ceremonial activities into the consumption of the beverage, originated in China. Tea began competing with romance as the inspiration for countless poems, songs and fine arts.

After the Tang Dynasty, tea plant seeds from China were spread into more than fifty countries. Today, tea is the most popular beverage in the world, with black tea accounting for 78 percent of the consumption and green tea most of the remainder. Tea production worldwide exceeds 2.9 million tons a year, with 80 percent produced in Asia. In the United States, tea consumption has increased 300 percent in ten years—the same time period that saw the country's first *decline* in per capita cancer rates.

So Prove It

Think we're on to something? I do, and for the past few years, I have set out to prove it.

Now, do not get me wrong. Science caught on to the healing properties of tea long before I came along, but I sensed there was much more to know. For the past fifteen years, my research has revolved almost exclusively around green tea because the more I learned, the more I found there *was* to learn. Once I learned about green tea's little army of chemicals that gobbles cancer cells, I learned about a complementary army that protects healthy cells. Then I learned that the chemicals can, astonishingly, regenerate skin cells and repair skin damage, including wrinkles and blemishes. Next was the finding that green tea helps protect against inflammation and autoimmune disease. Next came my growing fascination that there always seemed to be a *next.*

As a scientist, I am not easily shocked. By nature, I'm methodical, cautious and skeptical. Show me the result of a single experiment and I barely blink an eye. But demonstrate the same result again and again and again, and you have my attention. Confirm those results within intensely regulated scientific controls and I am pretty excited. Demonstrate that the same chemicals that help treat one disease can also help treat yet another—and another—and another—and I am blown away.

I am writing this book because, after years of conducting research in a methodical, cautious and skeptical way, I am now officially blown away. I wish you could visit my laboratory and see cancer cells in a Petri dish disappear after adding green tea. The results are truly that astonishing, and I want the world to know it. I want to confirm what Chinese folklore has been telling us for millennia. I want to tell you *why* green tea is healing, and *how,* and what it means for you and your family. I want to share my excitement because, frankly, it's a big deal when I get excited.

Most of all, I want you to live a long, healthy life, feel good and look good. Now, remember my original caveat: There are no magic pills. Green tea will not make you live forever, it will not make you super-model gorgeous and it will not keep you from spraining your ankle next time you go roller blading. But it *can* help you stay healthier and younger looking than you might have ever imagined, particularly now that green tea's healing properties are being incorporated into everyday products such as chewing gum, mints and skin care products (more about that later).

So heat yourself some water, pop in some tea leaves, curl up on the sofa and learn how what I have to tell you might just be your cup of tea.

Chapter II

What's in Your Cup of Tea?

Continental Divide

My adopted state of Georgia does not have an official beverage, but if it did, there is no doubt what it would be: sweet tea, loaded with sugar.

America was slower than Asia to warm to the charms of tea, but once iced tea was introduced at the World's Fair in St. Louis in 1904, the country—particularly the South—was hooked. When tea bags hit the scene four years later, Americans never looked back.

But until recently, tea in America had little in common with the green tea of my native culture. Now that a vast variety of teas including (hooray!) green teas commonly line the shelves of grocery stores throughout the United States, it is understandable if your head is swimming, wondering what differentiates one from another. Here is a crash course:

All Teas Are Not Created Equal

An evergreen shrub called the *Camellia sinesis* is the common origin of all teas. Tea bushes cultivated for harvest are generally around three feet tall. Experienced tea pickers collect up to 70 pounds of tea a day by hand, and one tea bush will produce tea for at least 50 years. A single pound of tea yields about 180 cups of brewed tea.

Tea boasts over 3,000 varieties, each with defining characteristics resulting from factors such as climate, soil and cultivation methods. Tea is harvested after the top two leaves and bud are hand-plucked, then processed into one of four types: black, green, oolong or white. (Herbal beverages, while packaged like teas, are made of grasses, barks, fruits, flowers and other botanicals that technically disqualify them as teas at all. But if you enjoy them, sip away. Just add *real* tea to your diet, too.)

Prior to cultivation, all teas share three properties: essential oils (the source of their aroma), caffeine (the stimulating property) and polyphenols—the wellness-packed compounds we will learn much more about later.

Black tea, by far the most popular variety in America, is crushed, withered, fermented and dried. As I noted, all teas, including black, have polyphenols, but black tea undergoes a complete oxidation process that neutralizes the compounds. Black tea still has many healthful properties, including several important minerals, but green tea trumps its cousin hands down in the wellness arena. Black tea produces a hearty, amber colored brew. Popular varieties include Keemen (the most famous black tea variety in China), English Breakfast and Darjeeling. Popular beverages in British tea shops, such as Earl Grey, are commonly blends of several fine black teas.

Oolong tea, popular in China, is crushed, withered, partially oxidized and dried. It brews pale green/golden with a delicate flavor. Originally grown in the Fujian province of China, it was the first imported to England in 1869 by John Dodd. Today, the highest-grade Oolongs (Formosa Oolongs) are grown in Taiwan. A cross between green and black teas, Oolong is semi-oxidized to achieve a fruity flavor.

White tea, the least processed, is a very rare tea from Fujian, China. This variety is from the budding leaves of tea plant. Rather than being oxidized or rolled, it is simply withered and dried. During the withering process, the polyphenols are briefly fermented, a process called micro fermentation. White tea tastes great because it is rich in amino acids. This tea shares the healthful properties of green tea but is much scarcer because of the limited availability of the budding leaves. A type of white tea from the Zhejiang province made from albino tea plants is even more rare and expensive. This brings us to the grand prize winner of healthful, inexpensive and widely available teas:

Green tea completely skips the oxidizing step and is simply heated, rolled and dried. The brief heating kills enzymes that would otherwise oxidize the polyphenols. The tea brews pale green/golden and has a delicate flavor that novices may perceive as slightly bitter, though it's easy to acquire a taste for the beverage.

Green tea does contain caffeine, from 2 to 5 percent, depending on the brand. However, a typical cup of green tea contains less than 30 milligrams of caffeine, compared to 100 milligrams in the average cup of coffee. The average person can easily tolerate this low level of caffeine, especially if you drink your green tea well before bedtime. Decaffeinated green tea is available for caffeine conscious consumers, but make sure your brand is decaffeinated using the "green" method of carbon dioxide rather than with caffeine extracting chemicals such as organic solvents. (Who wants to drink those? Yuck.) The decaffeination process may eliminate some polyphenols and detract from the aroma and flavor, but it is a worthy tradeoff if caffeine is definitely a no-no.

Bags Vs. Leaves

Green tea is sold both in bags and as loose leaves. I prefer the latter because I like minimal processing, but tea bags suit me fine in a pinch. My minimalist mentality also leads me to steer clear of green tea bags flavored with other ingredients, unless I'm sure the processing retained the healthful properties of the tea. For instance, I enjoy the wonderful aroma of green tea dried with jasmine flowers. But for the most part, my philosophy is that nature did a great job creating the tea leaf, and I am sticking as close to the original as possible.

When it comes to brands, I suggest cans or tins from oriental markets that tell you where and how the leaves were grown and processed. Once you are comfortable that you are getting the real (minimally processed) deal, let your taste buds lead the way when it comes to brands and kinds. Popular types include Dragon Well, Jasmine, Iron Buddha and Pearl.

Defining characteristics include:

- Aroma: the scent of the tea liquor, also called the nose or fragrance. A complex aroma is often called a bouquet.
- Astringency: The reaction between polyphenols and the protein in saliva.
- Body: The sensation of weight and substance experienced in the mouth.
- Fullness: Color, strength, substance and roundness.
- Thickness: Substance, but not necessarily strength.
- Strength: A range from thin and weak to thick and strong.

Organically Speaking

One caveat about my minimalist philosophy: I do not necessarily seek out organic green tea. Tea leaves do not attract a lot of insects, so they do not require a lot of pesticides. And the leaves grow on trees, which do not need constant fertilization. As a further precaution, tea products imported into the United States are generally tested to ensure acceptably low levels of heavy metals, pesticides, fertilizers and other chemicals. The Chinese government also cracks down hard on producers who do not meet high safety standards because tea is so vital to the country's economy. This is especially the case in Zhejiang province, where I buy my green tea each year in early spring. So in general, the green tea we drink is very safe. But if you eschew products that use *any* pesticide or chemical fertilizers, organic tea is a perfectly legitimate (though pricier) option. The challenge is how you would know this is a real organic tea. My definition of "organic farming" was before the invention of chemically synthesized fertilizers and pesticides, and in some places like in the Amazon rain forest.

Your Cup of Tea

What if, despite your healthiest intentions, your taste buds rebel at your decision to make green tea a regular part of your diet? Some of my American friends tell me they dislike the slightly bitter taste of green tea. All I can say is that most people who incorporate it into their diet come to genuinely enjoy the flavor, especially as a smooth, soothing, palate cleansing way to start the day. Asians particularly like the "second pour" of green tea, pouring hot water over the same leaves used for a first cup. Green tea tastes fresh and clean because that is just what it is. If it does not knock your socks off the first time you try it, hang in there. And if you *never* acquire a taste, keep drinking it and pat yourself on the back for doing something healthful in spite of your uncooperative taste buds.

I confess that I enjoy green tea so much, I have a hard time going without it. In 2006 I was in Prague for a scientific meeting. The weather was bitterly cold and I was desperate for a cup of hot green tea, but the beverage is not readily available in the Czech Republic. When I finally found a restaurant that served it (Da Tang, across from the Renaissance Hotel), I ate there every day, sometimes twice a day. Green tea is worth seeking out.

Still not sold? I recently partnered with CCA Industries, Inc., to develop gum and mints retaining all the healthful properties of green tea. A single mint or piece of Mega-T green tea gum delivers the health benefits of two cups of green tea. The products also taste terrific, are sugar- and caffeine-free and freshen your breath. What could be sweeter than that?

Cleared for Takeoff

Now that you are clear (as opposed to cloudy) on your green tea facts, it is time to begin our mission in earnest: cracking the code of green tea's most amazing secrets. I find it one of nature's truest forms of beauty that a single plant can hold such a multitude of benefits. Let's start learning what they are.

Chapter III

A Formidable Cancer Warrior

'It Can't Hurt'

When a colleague of mine at the Medical College of Georgia recently diagnosed a patient with a cancerous tongue lesion, she scheduled surgery to remove the lesion. Of course, this meant the patient would lose part of her tongue—a sad and often debilitating consequence of oral cancer.

The alternative—unchecked cancer growth—obviously was unthinkable, and the patient resigned herself to her fate. She agreed to return for surgery several weeks later.

It was almost an afterthought my colleague offered as the patient was leaving her office. "Why don't you start drinking green tea?" she suggested. "It can't hurt."

My colleague was familiar with my research and, while mildly skeptical of green tea's cancer fighting properties, felt the patient was entitled to any information that might help.

She could hardly contain her excitement when the patient returned for her surgery several weeks later. There was no lesion to remove. Her tongue was cancer free. She had taken her advice and begun drinking several cups of green tea a day.

It is hard to imagine a more dramatic result—but then, it is hard to imagine a heartier cancer fighter than green tea.

Declaring War on Cancer Cells

Properties in green tea not only declare war on cancer cells but place healthy cells in a state of suspended animation to protect them from friendly fire. This is a pretty remarkable finding. How does a humble little beverage manage such a mammoth achievement?

Remember the polyphenols I cited earlier as one of three components of green tea? Well, green tea polyphenols mean business. Their most powerful function seems to be their ability to help eliminate free radicals, which can combine with DNA to cause genes to mutate. If mutated genes slip under the radar of the defense system and cells with mutated genes proliferate uncontrollably, the result is cancer. Fewer free radicals mean a much lower cancer risk.

As if this was not dramatic enough, green tea polyphenols perform another amazing task: while targeting the cancer cells for destruction, they shuttle healthy cells to safety.

Green tea unleashes p-57, also called KIP2, a protein that helps regulate cell growth and differentiation. Elevated levels of p-57 suspend cell growth, in effect putting the cell to sleep. When p-57 levels return to normal, cell growth resumes.

In laboratory tests, my colleagues and I have determined that this state of suspended animation protects healthy cells from annihilation while spurring the death of cancerous cells. The cancer cells are killed quickly and specifically, and the healthy cells are left unharmed [1].

A Vital Juncture

Our next step was to trace the juncture where healthy cells are shuttled to safety and cancer cells are sentenced to death. We found that green tea polyphenols actually activate two separate pathways, one for normal cells and one for cancer cells. The polyphenols seem to serve as a sentinel, separating cells with p-57 from cancer cells, which lack p-57 [2].

Using human cancer cells, we found that while the normal cells are shuttled to safety, the polyphenols destroy the mitochondria of cancer cells. Mitochondria are the powerhouse of a cell, and a cell is very vulnerable without it. Once the mitochondria are destroyed, their contents activate a chemical called Capsase 3 as the trigger man that executes the weakened cell [3].

My slides of the process are very dramatic. Within forty-eight hours of being treated with green tea, oral cancer cells are virtually blighted, and normal cells are unaffected. My colleagues and I have further found that inserting cancer cells with the p-57 gene, which restores the vital protective protein they lack, spares them at least partially from destruction [4].

That one alteration changes the whole spectrum. In my lab tests, we genetically engineered tumor cells with activated p-57 gene. Only because we restored p-57, these tumor cells started to slow down and die, even without the presence of green tea. That is nothing short of amazing. More interestingly, when we transplanted these cancer cells with the p-57 gene in specially bred mice, these cells formed fewer or no tumors, indicating that green tea's function to elevate p-57 may help *prevent* cancer [5].

ROS on the Rise

And there is more great news. The seemingly most potent green tea polyphenol is a compound called EGCG. Armed with a National Cancer Institute grant, I found in 2003 that EGCG increases reactive oxygen species, or ROS, a form of oxidative stress in oral cancer cells. Cells with abnormally high levels of ROS become damaged. If the level is very high, the cells will be killed.

Environmental pollutants and normal cellular activities generate ROS, and the level can be raised by, for instance, excessive sun exposure. Many chemotherapeutic drugs work by increasing ROS to the point of killing cancerous cells. Unfortunately, cancer therapy typically cannot distinguish between normal and cancerous cells, so many healthy cells are caught in the crossfire.

My colleagues and I have found that adding EGCG to cells increases ROS levels in cancer cells but reduces them in healthy salivary gland and skin cells. All of our data indicate that EGCG can lower the ROS level of healthy cells and keep it low. This is very exciting because perhaps we can use EGCG to protect healthy cells after cancer treatment and prevent side effects that can cause patients to suffer all their lives [6].

For instance, oral cancer treatment can severely damage the salivary gland, impeding the ability to secrete saliva and resulting in a chronically dry mouth. What if the tumor cells can be killed without damaging the healthy cells that ensure adequate salivary secretion? EGCG seems to fill this role.

Breaking it Down

ROS, EGCG, p-57…. If your mind is swimming in alphabet soup right about now, let us break things down a bit. Here, at a glance, is how green tea fights cancer:

- Green tea helps eliminate cancer causing free radicals.
- It activates a protein that puts healthy cells to sleep, protecting them from harm while other compounds in green tea unleash an onslaught against cancer cells.
- Those compounds attack the mitochondria, or powerhouse, of cancer cells, rendering them weak and vulnerable.
- Green tea activates a molecule that deals the fatal blow to weakened cancer cells.
- Its compounds can help minimize or prevent some unpleasant and potentially debilitating side effects of cancer treatment.

Most of my work has involved oral cancer, but green tea has also proved remarkably effective against other kinds of tumors, including prostate, breast and cervical tumors. (See Chapter Eight for more exciting findings.)

And I cannot overstate the importance of a major breakthrough in oral cancer. The disease is nothing short of vicious, logging a stubbornly persistent 50 percent mortality rate. Approximately one American per hour loses his life to oral cancer, and many delay treatment until it is too late. The precancerous lesions, which look like white or red patches in the mouth, are not painful, so they are often ignored.

And even those who conquer oral cancer often pay a horrendous price, such as the loss of vital tissues. (Imagine life without a tongue or half the face.)

Those who use tobacco products are particularly at risk of oral cancer. I recommend that adults, particularly smokers, tobacco chewers and those with steady exposure to environmental carcinogens, slowly drink green tea several cups of green tea a day. The Mega-T gum and mints I created are other alternatives. The cancer fighting effects subside after several hours, so I recommend exposing the mouth to green tea every few hours.

And what if you already have oral cancer? All the more reason to start drinking it right away. When my colleague told her patient, “It can’t hurt,” she had no idea what an understatement that was. Now we know.

Actually, what we know just keeps growing. Eight years after publishing our hypothesis that green tea protects against oral cancer, a clinical study at the University of Texas MD Anderson Cancer Center showed improvement in 59 percent of people taking green tea extract to treat oral precancerous lesions, compared to 18 percent of study participants taking a placebo. If the scientific phrase “clinical response” strikes you as dry and boring, I invite you to look at before and after pictures of the study participants [7]. I am so glad to see even more validation of our hypothesis. Green tea is literally changing (and saving!) people’s lives.

References

[1] Hsu, S. (2001) Green Tea & Oral Cancer. *The Journal of Georgia Dental Association. 31*: 32-33.

[2] Hsu S., Lewis JE., Borke JL., Singh B., Dickinson DP, Caughman GB., Athar M., Drake L., Aiken AC., Huynh CT., Das B., Osaki T., and Schuster GS. (2001) Chemopreventive Effects of Green Tea Polyphenols Correlate with Reversible Induction of p57 Expression. *Anticancer Research. 21*: 3743-3748.

[3] Hsu S., Lewis J., Singh B., Schoenlein P., Osaki T., Athar M., Porter AG and Schuster G. (2002). Green Tea Polyphenol Targets the Mitochondria in Tumor Cells Inducing Caspase 3-Dependent Apoptosis. *Anticancer Research, 23*:1533-1540.

[4] Hsu S., Yu FS., Lewis J., Singh B., Borke J., Osaki T., Athar M and Schuster G. (2002) Induction of p57 Is Required for Cell Survival When Exposed to Green Tea Polyphenols. *Anticancer Research. 22*: 4115-4120.

[5] Yamamoto T, Digumarthi H, Aranbayeva Z, Wataha J, Lewis J, Messer R, Qin H, Dickinson D, Osaki T, Schuster G and Hsu S. Role of EGCG-targeted p57/KIP2 in reducing tumorigenicity of oral carcinoma cells and blocking c-jun N -terminal kinase-mediated apoptosis. *Toxicol Appl Pharmacol*. 2007 Nov 1;224(3):318-25.

[6] Yamamoto T, Hsu S, Lewis J, Wataha J, Ueta E, Osaki T, Luckwood P, Singh B, Dickinson D, and Schuster G (2003) . Green Tea Polyphenol

Causes Differential Oxidative Environments in Tumor versus Normal Cells. *J Pharmacol Exp Ther. 307*:230-6.
[7] Cancer Prevention Research, Dr. *Vassiliki Papadimitrakopoulo*, November 2009.

Chapter IV

MORE THAN SKIN-DEEP

HOW DO YOU LIKE THEM APPLES?

Let us imagine for a moment that you are holding a bruised apple. Those spongy brown spots make the apple pretty unappetizing. But before you take a bite, someone offers you a potion that can be applied to the brown spots, making the apple look shiny and lustrous. Now, mind you, the brown spots have not gone away. They just look better. But the apple is still damaged.

That is the concept of most skin care products on the market. They may do a fair job of covering up damaged skin, perhaps even simulating luster and dewiness. But the skin is still damaged.

Now suppose that the unappetizing apple could be restored to its bright red, crisp, sweet and juicy perfection. Suppose that instead of temporarily covering up skin damage, you could actually *heal* it.

Impossible, right? After all, skin has proven to be one of the most intractable organs to heal. Sun damage, pollution, environmental toxins and just the process of living take a toll on skin … and we wear the price tag every day of our lives. Nothing ages us more than our skin. We can dye our hair, tighten our abs, slim our thighs, whiten our teeth and perform a hundred other tasks to make ourselves look younger, but skin is a heartless truth teller. Even the radical solution of plastic surgery serves only to tighten the skin, not improve it. Adding to the problem is a sun worshipping culture that dooms us to look even older than our years.

Don't Throw in the Towel!

Ready to throw in the beach towel? Well, that is a start, and I certainly advocate limiting your sun exposure, with particular emphasis on protecting against cancer promoting sunburns. But that advice comes too late for many of us, and even those who wisely avoided sunbathing in our youth still probably have tell tale signs of skin damage such as wrinkles, uneven pigmentation, sallowness and sagginess.

So do we buy the products that, in effect, paint over the brown spots of a bruised apple? That was our only choice until recently.

No more.

As amazing as green tea's cancer fighting properties are, my colleagues and I have discovered something equally remarkable: green tea can breathe life back into dying skin cells.

Remember EGCG, the heavyweight champ of green tea polyphenols that helps protect us against cancer? My colleagues and I have found that it is just as powerful in improving our skin.

EGCG to the Rescue ... Again

My interest in the effects of green tea on the skin was sparked in 2001, when my wife gave birth to our first child, Alexander. Before we left the hospital, an elderly nurse advised my wife to place tea bags on her nipples if nursing caused irritation. Tea bags! I could not believe a health care professional would suggest a home remedy rather than some kind of polysyllabic drug in a tube.

I immediately began surfing the Internet to learn more and found reams of information about skin healing properties of tea. But hardly any of the information explained how or why it worked.

I did, however, stumble across papers by U.S. scientists describing the protective effect of green tea polyphenols against skin damage triggered by ultraviolet rays. Then I remembered an afterthought by my lab technician when I was studying oral cancer. She suggested adding green tea to lab samples of human skin cells to observe the results. I gave her the green light, but we were so busy with our cancer research that we forgot about the samples.

Until now. I went to my lab, revisited the skin samples and viewed the results in astonishment. The skin cells treated with green tea polyphenols showed much more energy than the untreated cells.

It seemed impossible. Skin cells have a highly predictable life cycle. As we know, the skin, the body's largest organ, is a semi permeable barrier protecting us from water loss and infections. But if that function sounds simple, trust me: It is not. We have to dig deeper to understand the remarkable complexity of how skin cells function.

A Study in Perpetual Motion

Skin consists of three portions: the epidermis (outer portion), dermis (mid-portion) and hypodermis (inner portion). The epidermis consists of four distinguishable layers of skin cells: the basal (bottom) layer, spinous layer, granular layer (mid-layer) and cornified (outer) layer.

Let's move from the bottom up.

Cells in the basal layer are responsible for constant cell division in order to supply young, undifferentiated skin cells, or keratinocytes, to the upper layers. When these young keratinocytes are pushed up by even younger cells from the basal layer, they start to show differences from the basal cells, such as the spiny structure characteristic of cells in the spinous layer. They also differentiate, making specialized proteins, keratins and other distinguishing characteristics, including lipids to form granules inside each cell.

The cells with granules form the granular layer. These cells continue to travel upward, and during the journey, they gradually lose the ability to divide. They also lose the cell nuclei and begin to stick to each other, forming a unique structure called the cornified envelope.

When this process is complete, the cells have died and piled up on the outer layer of the epidermis as flat sheets (the cornified layer). But these dead cells aren't just sitting there doing nothing. They are highly organized, flat sheets sealed by lipids and protein to form a structure like shingles on the roof. The "shingles" prevent water leakage and shield the body from bacteria and other environmental threats.

The whole process lasts about twenty-eight days. Sometimes, we can actually see the end point of this process in the form of skin flaking off the body.

That, in a nutshell, is the highly predictable and well documented life cycle of an epidermal skin cell. So how was it possible that I was now standing in my lab gazing at active, energetic skin cells in a Petri dish that should have died weeks earlier? I repeated the experiment and found, again, that skin cells treated with green tea polyphenols were still going strong when they should have died.

My wife's nurse knew anecdotally what I was witnessing in the lab: Tea soothes the skin because green tea polyphenols rejuvenate dying cells.

I immediately shared my test results with Dr. George Schuster, chairman of the Medical College of Georgia Department of Oral Biology and Maxillofacial Pathology (aka my boss at the time). He eagerly encouraged further research. My lab technician and I spent the next year growing millions of normal human skin cells, then treating some with green tea polyphenols and comparing them to the untreated cells.

A year into the research, the evidence was clear: the green tea polyphenols turned dying cells vital and active again.

A Fountain of Youth for Skin Cells

EGCG, that heavy hitting champ of polyphenols, seems to be a fountain of youth for skin cells. When exposed to EGCG, old cells in the upper layers of the epidermis start making new DNA again, a signal for cell division. More DNA means more energy. Reactivated and re-energized, the cells look better. As an added bonus, green tea polyphenols stimulate the cells to differentiate quickly, speeding their journey up to the top layer of skin so once they get there, the outer layer looks and functions better. In other words, the existing "shingles" stay in good shape for much longer, and top-notch reinforcements replace them before they have a chance to droop and wither.

My colleagues and I published the results of our research in 2003 in the *Journal of Pharmacology & Experimental Therapeutics*. Other groups were doing similar studies, but thanks to my wife's nurse, we were a small step ahead. Later, a group of scientists in Korea found that EGCG increases the thickness of skin and promotes skin cell growth in aged skin. Although it would be nice to make all the discoveries myself, I was thrilled by this development, not only because it supported and bolstered our findings but because it used human subjects rather than cells in a Petri dish.

I knew this was big. Really big.

It was becoming increasingly clear that it was possible to actually improve skin … not simply gloss over the damage.

The take-home message? Fill your swimming pool with green tea and take a plunge into the fountain of youth.

Well … not so fast.

An Absorbing Dilemma

In order to take advantage of green tea's skin healing properties, we need to deliver active green tea polyphenols into every skin layer of the epidermis. This is not easy because:

- Drinking green tea will not deliver adequate amounts of polyphenols into the skin
- Our skin is water proof and green tea polyphenols are water-soluble
- As very strong antioxidants, green tea polyphenols are not stable and are very easily oxidized if dissolved in water.

Ordinary skin care products made with these unstable green tea polyphenols do not work because they try to deliver the polyphenols by water, and skin is water-proof. I often wonder why people spend so much money on skin care products with all kinds of fruit and plant extracts, amino acids and other water-soluble compounds. The skin cannot absorb them, so the products can never really improve it.

What if the products claim to be "dermatologist recommended"? Well, the products *can* prevent water evaporation from your skin, which is a fine but very transient and superficial benefit. And oily stuff makes our skin look shinier and smoother, no doubt about that. (The potion painted on to the bruised apple … remember?) And products with plant derived antioxidants will help protect the top layer of our skin. But all these fixes are literally only skin-deep. They camouflage or temporarily moisturize the top layer of skin made of dead cells. But, back to our analogy, they never penetrate the red skin of the apple. I wanted to make the whole apple better to eliminate those pesky brown spots.

The Penetrating Truth

Since our skin barrier is made by lipids, lipid-soluble substances are easily absorbed. I was on a quest to formulize a product delivering the benefits of green tea polyphenols into the deep layers of the skin. But I am not a chemist, not a dermatologist, not even a polyphenol expert. I had more questions than answers. On the other hand, I have many contacts, colleagues and friends who are experts in these areas. I also have one advantage: I can read Chinese very well, even in some chemistry terms.

Dr. Xian Qiang Yang, a professor at the Tea Research Institute in China, is one of the most respected green tea researchers in China and a prolific writer on the subject. One of his books, *The Chemistry of Tea Polyphenols,* has rich knowledge on the chemistry of polyphenols. Dr. Ping Chen, also a professor in the institute, is a chemistry genius who published some papers in Chinese that we cannot find here in the United States. When I contacted them, they warmly welcomed me to China.

Suddenly, I was back in my home country, talking sometimes until 2 a.m. with my new friends and colleagues about the plant that I had grown decades earlier on the 53rd Farm. We discussed all aspects of the beneficial properties of green tea and possible ways to utilize it to improve health. I felt enlightened and energized when I returned to my lab.

An Entrepreneur is Born

After more meetings and discussions with experts worldwide about key issues regarding polyphenols, I sat down in my office, read more books and studied the ingredients of many skin care products. I felt it was time to carry the information beyond the confines of my lab.

I was not the only one. Because of my publications and lectures, word was starting to get around about my green tea research. But I assumed the interest was confined to the scientific community. I assumed wrong.

I was working in my office when my secretary transferred a phone call from Malcolm Julian representing CCA Industries, Inc. I had never heard of him or the company, but he had heard of me and wanted to meet. He invited me to the company's headquarters in New Jersey, where he proposed partnering to create skin care products that retain the healing benefits of green tea.

The timing was perfect. As I noted earlier, other skin care products claim to have green tea benefits, but I knew enough now to understand why they did not work … and how I could create products that *did.* I partnered with CCA Industries to create a unique formulation in which green tea polyphenols are embedded in lipid, not water. Since they are not exposed to oxygen (which a water mixture would necessitate), the products are very stable, even in extremely hot weather. And since they are carried by lipids, they easily penetrate the skin barrier.

Thus, unlike any other green tea containing skin care product, our formulation (now available in products called the Sudden Change line) enables green tea polyphenols to be stable, active and permeable through every skin layer.

The result is not healthier *looking* skin. It is *healthier* skin. My green tea skin care products revitalize the skin cells, in effect turning back the clock. Rickety old cells are now replaced quickly by youngsters ready to take on the world.

'I Couldn't Believe My Eyes'

Independent dermatologists have since confirmed the products' effectiveness [1]. One study notes that within twenty-four hours, 75 percent of subjects improved in at least one characteristic of aged or damaged skin (for instance, wrinkles and lack of elasticity). After a week, wrinkles, fine lines, elasticity, texture and complexion were improved in *one hundred percent* of study participants. Not a single adverse effect was reported.

The independent dermatologists concluded that the results were "promising, effective and efficient for facial rejuvenation," noting "visible improvement in facial skin after twenty-four hours."

I have to admit that as convinced as I was of the products' effectiveness, this report surprised even me. Results in *twenty-four hours*? Improvement in *a hundred percent* of study participants? I called one of the dermatologists who conducted the study, just to make sure my eyes were not deceiving me. When she realized who was calling, she said just two words: "It worked." Eager for still more verification (I am a scientist, remember?) I called her colleague and asked, "Do you mean twenty-four hours?"

He responded, "Twenty-four hours. I couldn't believe my eyes."

More Good News

As exciting as these results are, the news only gets better. We all want to look youthful and healthy, and I am thrilled to have helped create a new means to that end. But the skin can harbor much greater danger than wrinkles and blemishes. As the body's largest organ, and the organ most vulnerable to the assaults of daily living, the skin can play havoc with our health. Some skin diseases can even kill us.

So can green tea not only make us look younger, but help treat skin diseases? The answer is yes. Let us move on to the next chapter to find out how.

References

[1] July 8, 2005 clinical evaluation of Skin Fit for Life Skin Cell Serum on facial rejuvenation, by Dr. Dan Chalker.

Chapter V

DIGGING DEEPER

FLAKE, FLAKE, FLAKE

I am a basic scientist, as opposed to a clinical scientist, which means my research takes place in a lab. I have wonderful colleagues who can take my results to the next step by testing them on patients, but early in the process, my work is a solitary affair.

That is why when an idea struck me recently, I decided to make myself a guinea pig.

Time for a confession: I have dandruff. (Well, technically, I *had* dandruff. Read on.) In the scheme of things, this is not a big deal, but it certainly caused me a fair share of discomfort and embarrassment.

The condition—an autoimmune response that causes an overproduction of cells, resulting in a dry, flaky scalp—affects fully a quarter of the human race, so dandruff shampoos have always been in hot demand, including by me. But I hated dandruff shampoos, which generally use coal tar to treat the damaged scalp. *Coal tar*. The stuff is a known carcinogen. Benzo(a)pyrine is the active ingredient in most dandruff shampoos, and that particular element of coal tar is a particularly nasty carcinogen.

We generally associate carcinogens with things we put into our bodies (tar is a cigarette ingredient, for instance), but environmental carcinogens take their toll, too, and I want to minimize my exposure to cancer causing elements as much as possible. On the other hand, coal tar definitely does control overproduction of cells, so it generally works to control dandruff and psoriasis.

But rather than choose between dandruff (which I hate) and coal tar (which in addition to being a carcinogen also smells awful), I wondered if I could create a better alternative. By this point, I learned how green tea polyphenols can rejuvenate dying skin cells and speed the process of healthy cells replacing their dying counterparts. Surely, those findings had implications for my dandruff … or was that just wishful thinking?

I decided to find out.

Washing That Dandruff Right Out of My Hair

I took the lipid bound green tea polyphenols, mixed them with different oils and detergent, then combined the concoction with a bottle of regular shampoo. I washed my hair with it twice a day … and in a week, my dandruff was gone. No more flakes. No more itchy scalp.

After a week, I began shampooing just once a day, and my dandruff is a thing of the past.

Of course, one experiment falls far short of the rigorous demands of good science, but I was fascinated enough by the results to dig deeper.

Assuming the shampoo was the cause of my new and improved scalp (at this point, that was just an assumption, albeit an educated assumption), how did it work? And might it work on other skin diseases? It was time to find out.

As we noted in Chapter Four, the skin, as the body's largest organ, is vulnerable to many genetic and environmental assaults. It is also the organ where those assaults are most noticeable. Skin conditions aren't only unhealthy, they're potentially embarrassing and can create considerable emotional pain.

Let us take a look at some common skin diseases:

Psoriasis

Psoriasis, one of those unfortunate autoimmune diseases referenced earlier, is likely a genetic condition that affects the skin and/or joints. Affecting 4.5 million Americans, the disease can range from mild to severe. The most common type, plaque psoriasis, causes patches called lesions, which become inflamed and covered by silvery white scales that can be limited to small areas or cover large areas of skin.

Remember when I talked about the average life cycle of a skin cell? Skin cells originate in the innermost skin layer, then migrate toward the surface of the skin where they begin dying, then slough off. This process in healthy skin takes about twenty-eight days. But in psoriasis, skin cells take only three to four days to mature and move to the surface. Instead of falling off, cells pile up and form lesions.

Forms of psoriasis include plaque, the most common type; guttate, characterized by small dot-like lesions; pustular, characterized by weeping lesions and intense scaling; inverse, characterized by intense inflammation; and erthyrodermic, characterized by intense shedding and redness. In all cases, the disease is uncomfortable, causing itchy skin when chemicals stimulate nerve fibers within the skin.

Psoriasis usually appears around ages fifteen to thirty-five, but it can strike at any age. Triggers for outbreaks include stress, skin injury, some types of infection and reactions to drugs. Itchy skin arises when chemicals stimulate nerve fibers within the skin.

Rosacea

This facial disorder affecting fourteen million American is characterized by facial redness, bumps, pimples and eye irritation. The disease is chronic and affects more women than men, typically showing up after age thirty.

The disease has four subtypes, and the condition evolves from one subtype to another in seventy-two percent of patients with the disease. Seventy-seven percent experience more than one subtype at the same time. Here is a breakdown:

- Subtype 1: Suffered by eighty-three percent, this subtype causes facial redness and, in some cases, visible blood vessels.
- Subtype 2: Affecting sixty-two percent, this subtype results in facial redness, bumps and pimples.
- Subtype 3: Affecting fifteen percent, this subtype causes skin thickening, usually on nose.
- Subtype 4: Affecting fifty percent, this subtype results in eye irritation.

Those with blonde hair and blue eyes at higher risk for rosacea, but the condition can affect any skin type. Triggers for outbreaks include hot drinks, spicy foods, caffeine and alcohol; excessive sun exposure; rubbing, scrubbing and massaging the face; exercise in hot weather; and some cosmetic products, including hair spray.

Wounds

Of course, everyone can (and does) suffer wounds to the skin, and the body usually does a magnificent job repairing the damage. But those with diabetes, compromised immune systems and/or conditions that can make it hard to change body positions can suffer terribly from seemingly harmless scratches, bruises and scrapes.

For these people, wounds can hang on tenaciously and resist healing. One of the most important roles of the skin is to serve as a barrier against infection and other environmental assaults, so skin that does not heal is very vulnerable to infection. The results—including amputations for diabetics and bed sores for bedridden patients—can be terribly painful and debilitating. Also, if skin cells surrounding wounds or infections do not heal in time, fibroblasts in the connective tissue may rush in to fill the void and cause scar tissue formation.

Controlling the Pace

All of these skin conditions have something in common, other than the suffering they cause: the skin cells are differentiating at abnormal rates, disturbing the normal skin cell cycle and leaving traces of their damage for all the world to see. What if we could control the pace of the skin cell differentiation? As we learned in the Chapter Four, we can … with EGCG.

I am tremendously excited about the potential of developing green tea products (lotions, shampoos, detergents and more) to help normalize a diseased process of skin cell differentiation. For instance, if we can accelerate the wound healing process, we can help prevent scarring and infection. If we can slow the overgrowth of skin cells, we can tackle diseases such as psoriasis and, the bane of my existence, dandruff.

This research is in its infancy, but now that we realize the ability of EGCG to revitalize dying cells and spur the differentiation process, we have opened the door to a whole new world of potential to battle skin diseases*.

* The skin diseases I have cited are those I feel have the most promise in responding to green tea polyphenols. There are others, of course, including the nightmare of teens everywhere: acne. Although it is clear that green tea can improve anyone's skin condition, acne has an added element—bacteria—that would probably necessitate an added antibacterial component in order for green tea products to target blemishes.

Chapter VI

FAT CHANCE

FOOD FOR THOUGHT

You can tell a lot about a culture from its advertisements.

In my native country, China, most television commercials are about skin care products and medications. In my adopted country, the United States, most are about food, drinks and cars. My tongue-in-cheek theory is that manufacturers want us to eat until we are so fat that we cannot walk anymore … at which point it is time to buy a car. (Okay, maybe it is not so tongue-in-cheek.)

But there is nothing funny about obesity. As the nutrition course director at the Medical College of Georgia, I am all too aware of the alarming situation in our country: 66 percent of adult Americans are overweight and 34 percent are obese, according to the U.S. Centers for Disease Control and Prevention. Obesity is now categorized as a disease by the government. And it is not just a sickness … it is an epidemic.

As recently as 1996, not a single state in the country had an obesity rate of over 20 percent. Today, fully forty-nine of the country's fifty states exceed that level. (Kudos to the lone holdout: Colorado.)

What does this mean for our health? Loosen your belt buckle so you can take a deep breath as you read this sobering list of obesity related diseases [1]:

- Hypertension
- Dyslipidemia (for example, high total cholesterol or high levels of triglycerides)
- Type 2 diabetes

- Coronary heart disease
- Stroke
- Gallbladder disease
- Osteoarthritis
- Sleep apnea
- Respiratory problems
- Some cancers (endometrial, breast, and colon)

Among theses diseases, diabetes and cardiovascular disease are particularly problematic. The latter is the most deadly, and the incidence of type 2 diabetes has exploded nationally. Potential complications of diabetes, including blindness and circulation problems that can require limb amputation, cause a massive amount of disability, and at increasingly young ages.

Unum Provident Corporation, the nation's largest provider of disability income protection insurance, reports that obesity related disability claims have increased tenfold over the past decade. The company also says that patients with obesity related disabilities have significantly higher medical costs than those with other types of disabilities, averaging more than $51,000 a year. According to Unum, obesity related disabilities cost employers about $8,720 per employee per year, not counting direct medical costs of $30,567 [2].

A Pain in the Pocketbook

Of course, those medical bills, disability payments and loss of productivity affect the economy for all of us, whether or not we are overweight. And the pain in our pocketbooks does not end there. Medical expenses for obesity related illnesses account for about 10 percent of all U.S. medical costs, a figure approaching $100 billion a year. Half of that figure comes from Medicare and Medicaid—in other words, from you and me, the taxpayers [3]. That's right, folks: $50 billion of our tax dollars are spent treating obesity related diseases alone.

Care for a bit of context? The National Institutes of Health, the organization responsible for all government funded medical research in this country, has an annual budget of about $30 billion a year. Just imagine the strides we could make—the diseases we could cure and the suffering we could end—if we could spend an extra $50 billion on biomedical research rather than on treatments for obesity related problems.

As dire as these statistics are, the saddest is the fact that the obesity epidemic has now engulfed our children. The U.S. Centers for Disease Control and Prevention recently reported that the number of overweight youth has more than tripled since 1980. Among those ages 6-19, sixteen percent (over nine million) are considered overweight.

It is sometimes hard to tease out the contributions of genetics and environment when tackling a disease. But when numbers jump this dramatically in so brief a time span, the culprit is clear: environment. We are fat because we are eating too much and exercising too little.

Try, Try Again

We have tried pretty much everything to reverse the course. But the failure of one diet after another only demonstrates the futility of that course. Weight maintenance should not be a constant battle; it should be a happy side effect of a peaceful, healthful existence.

Consider the recent Atkins diet, encouraging over-consumption of meat and fat and under-consumption of fruits, vegetables and grains. (Our noble friend, the carbohydrate, got a terribly undeserved rap during this craze.) Did the diet work? No, chiefly because both the individual dieter and his body eventually rebelled against such unnatural eating habits. The Atkins industry recently declared bankruptcy.

Another tool in our ever growing obesity arsenal is surgery. Stomach stapling, fat sucking and intestine-removing procedures indicate the depths of our desperation to be thin. Cutting, slicing, suctioning, stapling … we know intuitively that these "solutions" cannot possibly be healthy for any except the morbidly obese who might die without fast and drastic action.

And again, we are left with the glum reality that, even with all these tools at our disposal, we are fatter than ever. It only makes sense to look at lean populations, then compare and contrast.

Time for East to Meet West

The United States, the United Kingdom and Australia: These are wonderful countries (as I can personally attest) with countless admirable attributes. But they share the unfortunate statistic of 20-plus percent obesity rates, compared to a 3 percent obesity rate in Japan [4]. Many factors are involved, but I think it is a mistake to overcomplicate this issue. Let's use our common sense (now bolstered by hard science) to help determine why we are so much fatter than the Japanese.

First, let's consider what Japan and the United States have in common. Both are developed countries, so both populations have access to all kinds of food. Both countries are more sedentary than they should be. Japan, which makes more cars per capita than any country in the world, is not averse to guzzling gasoline. The country is small, so the Japanese are much more confined than Americans and have fewer exercise facilities. If you go to Japan, you will find people playing golf in a small room in front of a simulated golf course on a big screen TV. Membership to a real golf course in Japan can cost tens of thousands of dollars.

So common denominators of Japan and the United States include a vast array of food choices and a relatively sedentary lifestyle. Yet our obesity rate is still ten times that of Japan's.

And what about my native country, China? The obesity rate is around 7 percent. The Chinese are far more active than the average American, most lack cars and walk or ride bicycles everywhere they go. But since the introduction of fast food chains to China around a decade ago, the average Chinese diet has become high in calories, fat and sugar—and the obesity rate has doubled [5]. NBA star Yao Ming has partnered with McDonald's to hasten the spread of American "progress" to his home country. I wrote an article for the Chinese *Hospital Newspaper* fifteen years ago warning the population about two risks: obesity and the AIDS epidemic. My warnings were largely ignored, and the Chinese are paying the price.

So we see that food choices in Asia are not necessarily healthy, and the Japanese are not much more active than we are. But their obesity rates are far, far lower. The most consistent variable I can find is green tea. Asians drink it regularly, and most Americans do not. Can one little beverage really tip the scales so dramatically?

Forty Pounds Ago

If you had met me in 1988 and asked when I moved to the United States, I would have joked, "Forty pounds ago."

I was an undergraduate student in 1982 when I ate my first Big Mac in Iowa during a snowstorm. I remember thinking, "This tastes so different from Chinese food!" Accompanied with an ice cold Coke and golden french fries, I had embarked on my first truly American meal. And I liked it. Actually, I loved it. But luckily, I didn't have enough money at the time to buy much fast food, so my waistline remained intact until I began a full time Ph.D. program in Cincinnati. With a generous scholarship and help from my Uncle Henry, Big Macs were suddenly within my price range. I often had a Value Meal for lunch: Big Mac, fries and Coke, plus an ice cream sundae with chocolate fudge. My overweight classmate, David, always joined me. Green tea was not on the menu.

Further hastening my Americanization was my newly acquired sedentary lifestyle. Because of my extensive coursework, my exercise consisted of one to three hours of basketball a week. Within six years of my new lifestyle, my weight had risen to 180 pounds. My girlfriend (now my wife, Tracy) warned me, "If you keep drinking gallons and gallons of Coke, you will eventually turn Coke colored."

Now, I am not going to vouch for the science behind Tracy's prediction, but I am proud to say I was smart enough to heed her warning anyway. I eliminated soft drinks from my diet, began drinking more green tea and started playing basketball at least three times a week with my students. Today, I maintain a healthy weight in the 160s and still play competitive sports well into my fifties. I had learned firsthand how quickly a healthy lifestyle can slip away, and to this day, I am thankful to my wife for urging me to make corrections.

So I know plenty about both Asian and American lifestyles. Let's take a look at the science that explains how the world has become divided into the East (the lean) and the West (the fat).

Back to the Lab

Scientists in the food industry admit that typical diets do not work and recommend exploring new dietary components, including green tea [6].

Japanese scientists recently conducted a study feeding two groups of rats a diet rich in fats and sugar, supplementing the diet of one group with green tea. They found that the rats that consumed green tea had fewer fat deposits in the body and lower blood cholesterol than the other rats [7]. In a European study using rats, two groups were fed high-fat, high-cholesterol food for four months; one group was also fed EGCG, the powerful polyphenol in green tea that I have talked about at length. The group with EGCG showed significantly lower cholesterol and LDL levels, a measure of the absorption of cholesterol and fat in the blood [8].

A very sophisticated American study showed the same result. These scientists infused cholesterol with or without green tea extract into two groups of rats, and found green tea blocked the intestinal absorption of cholesterol [9]. If cholesterol was not absorbed, where did it go? A Chinese team in Hong Kong answered this question by testing rats consuming cholesterol and green tea. They reported that rats fed with Dragon Well green tea (my favorite) absorbed much less cholesterol but excreted more in the feces [10]. Similar results were obtained from another study using mice. These results indicated that lipid metabolism in mice was suppressed by administering green tea, thereby suppressing fatty accumulation and weight gain [11].

JUST A FAD?

At this point, I am guessing some skepticism may be creeping in. "Sure, there's evidence supporting how green tea can help maintain a healthy weight," you may be thinking, "but I've heard other reports claiming that green tea is just a fad."

For instance, a researcher interviewed on the ABC news magazine, *20-20,* said tests on rats are basically meaningless because rodents' metabolism differs from that of humans. (She did not convince the show's host, incidentally; beautiful Elizabeth Vargas drinks green tea regularly.)

And yes, test results on rats are not necessarily meaningful for humans. But if that logic kept us from conducting animal studies, we would still be plagued with countless diseases and sources of suffering that we eliminated with research that began with animal studies. To discount green tea studies just because the study models are rats is to discount study results that eventually yielded countless cures and treatments.

But other researchers have echoed skepticism about health benefits of green tea, so I will indulge them by saying, "Okay, fellas. You're on. You've set the bar awfully high to insist that only *human* studies count, but so be it."

The benefits of green tea withstand even *this* stringent criterion. In 1999, a group of scientists at the University of Geneva reported their *human* clinical trial using either green tea extract or placebo. Their result suggests that "the green tea extract may play a role in the control of body composition via sympathetic activation of thermogenesis, fat oxidation, or both" [12]. To make it simple: green tea helps you burn more fat.

This was an extremely well controlled study, using three groups of human subjects with one group consuming a placebo, one group consuming the green tea extract and one group consuming the caffeine in the amount found in the green tea extract. By designing the study this way, the researchers eliminated the caffeine factor. Actually, caffeine failed to burn more fat in that study. Three years later, a French team of researchers reached the same conclusion that green tea extract helps burn more fat. They also found that green tea extract inhibited enzymes that digest fat. More importantly, they found that after three months of green tea extract consumption, obese patients showed, on average, 4.6 percent weight loss and 4.5 percent waist reduction [13].

Now, on to the cholesterol business: a research team at Vanderbilt University Medical Center reported in 2003 that green tea extract lowered total blood cholesterol by 11 percent and LDL by 16 percent, while the placebo group didn't show any change. This was a human clinical trial, also well controlled, with 240 adult patients with mild or moderate high cholesterol [14]. In 2005, a group of Japanese scientists reported in the *American Journal of Nutrition* that healthy men of similar age and body weight were asked to consume an identical diet for two weeks except for one variable: green tea. One group drank enough green tea daily to consume 690 milligrams of polyphenols. The other group drank enough to consume 22 milligrams of polyphenols. After twelve weeks, body weight, body mass index waist circumference, body fat mass, cholesterol (in a form of oxidized LDL) and subcutaneous fat were significantly lower in the group consuming 690 milligrams [15].

A similar study with healthy subjects in Italy, where almost no one drinks green tea, showed the group consuming 250 milligrams of green tea polyphenols per day for 42 days decreased cholesterol by more than 10 percent. In addition, the green tea group demonstrated much more antioxidant activity in the blood [16].

As scientists, we must rely on evidence. In this case, we need to look at the evidence from molecules, proteins, DNA and RNA, then move on to genes—thousands of genes—before moving on to cells, all different kinds of cells, before moving on to animal studies, then finally human studies. To either affirm or discount research results prematurely is to not only embarrass ourselves, but to mislead the public.

So I welcome skepticism. And I am proud to present the growing body of hard science that answers that skepticism so decisively.

How Much of a Good Thing?

Now that it is clear green tea helps maintain a healthy weight while lowering cholesterol and LDL levels, you are no doubt wondering how to incorporate green tea into your diet for optimal results.

I touched briefly on ways to incorporate green tea into your diet in Chapter Two, but let's get more specific at this point. Is it safe to drink a lot?

MD Anderson Cancer Center, one of the most prestigious cancer centers in the United States, conducted a human study on green tea consumption several years ago. Researchers concluded it is safe to drink the equivalent of seven to eight Japanese cups of green tea three times a day [17]. The only health concern was caffeine consumption, a concern precluded by caffeine free green tea products such as gum and mints.

Another clinical trial showed that it is safe for healthy individuals to consume green tea polyphenol products in amounts equivalent to the EGCG content in eight to sixteen cups of green tea daily, or in divided doses twice a day for four weeks [18]. For the purified form of green tea polyphenols, either in EGCG form or in a combination of all polyphenols, a single dose of up to 0.8 grams was found to be completely safe. The blood polyphenols increased after the consumption and peaked four hours later.

However, the blood level was found to contain only a fraction of the amount consumed. Why is that? Scientists think humans have a mechanism to block excessive amounts of polyphenolic compounds from entering the blood stream. An excess may cause proteins to bind in the blood, so this "natural" barrier prevents any harmful interactions.

If the extensive citations of scientific studies in this chapter have you seeing double at this point, I apologize. But I think it is vital to have at least a casual familiarization of the science behind the claims, particularly since green tea has become such a target for those crying foul, rip off, scam or fad. No one hates bad science or pseudoscience more than I do, and I will be the first one to expose any such examples. Aren't you glad, for your waistline's sake, that green tea has been so thoroughly researched, and has passed the tests with flying colors?

Now we understand why Oprah, who is from the southern state of Mississippi, is a big fan of green tea. She doesn't endorse beef steaks, barbecue ribs, sweet tea, hot dogs, ice cream, fries, hamburgers or even apple pie. Nope … she endorses green tea!

References

[1] U.S. Centers for Disease Control and Prevention
[2] Unum Provident Corporation news release, Feb. 17, 2004
[3] U.S. Centers for Disease Control and Prevention
[4] Organization for Economic Co-operation and Development Health Policy Unit, September 2003.
[5] Forbes Magazine, "Fat in China" by Dan Ackman, Oct. 13, 2004
[6] Critical Review of Food and Science Nutrition, "A functional food product for the management of weight," S.J. Bell and G.K. Goodrick, March 2002.
[7] Phytotherapy., "Powdered green tea has antilipogenic effect on Zucker rats fed a high-fat diet," N. Hasegawa, N. Yamda and M. Mori, May 2003.
[8] In Vivo, "Effects of green tea on growth, food utilization and lipid metabolism in mice," K. Sayama, S. Lin, G. Zheng and I. Oguni, July-August 2000.
[9] *Journal of Nutrition and Biochemistry*, "Effects of EGCG on lipid absorption and plasma lipid levels in rats," D.G. Raederstorff, M.F. Schlachter, V. Elste and P. Weber, June 2003.
[10] *Journal of Nutrition*, "Green tea extract inhibits the lymphatic absorption of cholesterol and alpha-tocopherol in ovariectomized rats," H.B. Loest, S.K. Noh and S.I. Koo, June 2002.
[11] *Life Science*, "Chinese green tea lowers cholesterol level through an increase in fecal lipid excretion," T.T. Yang and M.W. Koo, June 2000.
[12] *American Journal of Clinical Nutrition*, "Efficacy of a green tea extract rich in catechin polyphenols and caffeine in increasing 24-hour energy expenditure and fat oxidation in humans," A.G. Dulloo, C. Duret, D.

Roher, L. L. Girardier, N. Mensi, M. Fathi, P. Chantre and J. Vandermander, December 1999.

[13]*Phytomedicine* « Recent findings of green tea extract AR25 (Exolise) and its activity for the treatment of obesity, » P. Chantre and D. Lairon, January 2002.

[14]*Archives of Internal Medicine*, "Cholesterol-lowering effect of a theaflavin-enriched green tea extract: a randomized controlled trial," D.J. Maron, G.P. Lu, N.S. Cai, Z.G. Wu, Y.H. Li, H. chen, J.Q. Zhu, X.J. Jin, B.C. Wouters and J. Zhao, June 2003.

[15]*American Journal of Clinical Nutrition*, "Ingestion of a tea rich in catechins leads to a reduction in body fat and malondialdehyde-modified LDL in men," T. Nagao, Y. Komine, S. Soga, S. Meguro, T. Hase, Y. Tanaka and I. Tokimitsu, January 2005.

[16]*Clinical Cancer Research*, "Pharmacokinetics and safety of green tea polyphenols after multiple-dose administration of epigallocatechin gallate and polyphenon E in healthy individuals," H.H. Chow, Y. Cai, I.A. Hakim, J.A. Crowell, F. Shahi, C.A. Brooks, R.T. Dorr, Y. Hara and D.S. Alberts, August 2003.

[17]*Journal of Clinical Oncology*, "Phase 1 trial of oral green tea extract in patients with solid tumors," K.M. Pisters, R.A. Newman, B. Coldman, D.M. Shin, F.R. Hkuri, W.K. Hong, B.S. Glisson and J.S. Lee, March 2001.

[18]*Cancer Epidemiological Biomarkers Preview*, "Phase I pharmacokinetic study of tea polyphenols following single-dose administration of epigallocatechin gallate and polyphenon E," H.H. Chow, Y. Cai, D.S. Alberts, I. Hakim, R. Dorr, F. Shahi, J.A. Crowell, C.S. Yang, Y. Hara, January 2001.

Chapter VII

ASSAULT WEAPON

A WHOLE NUTHER BALL OF WAX

Remember the skin conditions, such as dandruff and psoriasis, that I referenced in Chapter Five? Many of them belong to a big disease group: autoimmune diseases, the third largest category of diseases in the country, after heart diseases and cancer. There are more than sixty-five types affecting eight percent of the U.S. population—a whopping 25 million people. Each year, we spend approximately $120 billion treating these diseases.

Few conditions have stymied the medical community through the ages as much as autoimmune diseases.

While no disease is pleasant, some are relatively straightforward and easy to understand: A cell divides more than it should and creates cancer. A weakened heart ceases to pump efficiently and causes a heart attack. Plaque filled arteries impede blood flow and prompt a stroke.

Tragic yet understandable.

Autoimmune diseases, on the other hand, are (to borrow a phrase common in my adopted homeland of America's Deep South) a whole nuther ball of wax.

At its simplest level, an autoimmune disease involves the body attacking itself. Different autoimmune diseases involve different targets—for instance, rheumatoid arthritis involves the joints, type 1 diabetes the pancreas, multiple sclerosis the central nervous system, psoriasis the skin, etc.—but the common denominator is the body assaulting itself. It defies the most basic logic; the immune system is supposed to *protect* the body, not assault it.

When that happens, everything changes: the body mobilizes for a big war—against its own tissues and organs yet!

A Formidable Army

Let's take a closer look at the immune system to analyze precisely what's going on:

No army is of much use without weapons, and the immune system has one of the most impressive arsenals you will ever find.

That arsenal comes in the form of a specialized set of cells: lymphocytes, also called white blood cells. Each cell population comprises a specialized force. For example, B cells produce antibodies. When B cells receive messages from other immune cells (T cells and macrophages), the alarm sounds and they start dividing like crazy, producing a huge amount of antibody against a piece of molecule with precise accuracy. Soon, the antibodies are coursing through the bloodstream, attacking any cell with the targeted molecule.

And those T cells that alerted the B cells in the first place? A subgroup of them, appropriately called T killer cells, are even *more* vicious. They leave the bloodstream entirely to target tissues, organs and cells with the offending molecule. Another subgroup, T helper cells, amplifies the immune reaction by alarming other cell populations and guiding them to the targets.

Finally, yet another group of white blood cells rushes to the scene and gobbles the target to pieces. Adding insult to injury, the cells feed some of those pieces to T helper cells and B cells for more reinforcement and attacks until the war is finally over.

Ouch!

As violent and unsettling as these war games may sound, they serve us well—*when* the offending molecules represent bacteria or viruses that can hurt us. But when they are our own tissues? That is not war, that is suicide! At least at the molecular level.

Every year, the National Institutes of Health spends tens of millions dollars trying to determine what triggers these misguided attacks. Many pieces of the puzzle are still missing, but we're learning more and more all the time. And wouldn't you know it? We are learning how green tea can help. (Ahhhh . . . back to green tea!)

Read My Lips

Let's focus for a moment on one autoimmune disease in particular: Sjogren's syndrome. This disease prompts the immune system to attack the glands that produce tears and saliva, causing unnaturally dry eyes and mouth. Sjogren's isn't the *only* cause of dry mouth (more than 400 medications, radiation therapy and other diseases like diabetes can also cause it), but it is a *major* cause, and a major problem. Almost a third—yes, a *third*—of elderly Americans suffer from dry mouth, and Sjogren's is incurable.

"Unfortunate," you may be thinking, "but if it is an age related condition—well, old people get sick. It is just a regrettable fact of life."

Not so fast. The fact that fully a third of elderly Americans suffer from dry mouth, or xerostamia, may suggest a natural wear-and-tear process. But hop across the ocean to my home country of China and you will realize there is nothing inevitable about dry mouth at all. Fewer than five percent of elderly Chinese suffer from the problem. Five percent compared to thirty percent? By this point, I should not have to tell you what I deduced when I learned this statistic.

But I will anyway.

I suspected the answer lay in green tea.

The Chinese, as we have established, typically consume several cups of green tea a day throughout most of their lives. Only recently has the drink become popular in the United States, and even now, it is not nearly as entrenched in the Western lifestyle, particularly among seniors, as it is in the East. I know very few elderly Americans who drink green tea regularly, if at all.

We have already definitively established that green tea helps protect tissues with which it comes in direct contact. Salivary glands are embedded deep within the mouth. Does green tea help protect *them?* And if so, how?

Back to the lab.

Un-SS-B-lievable!

It was a cold afternoon early in 2004. (Yes, even balmy Augusta, Georgia has its share of cold days!) My colleague, Dr. Carol Lapp, came to my office carrying a computer generated sheet with one line highlighted in neon yellow. On the right side of the line, a symbol caught my eye: SS-B.

Dr. Lapp and I had been researching green tea's effect on tumors and skin disease, following lots of exciting leads. Our research included analyzing the entire human genome, determining which genes and their associated proteins reacted to the chemicals in green tea.

SS-B is one of those proteins, but I never expected it to be a player in our research. The protein performs a normal role in most cells to help with RNA functions. But it is also a major target for autoantibodies in patients with lupus or Sjogren's syndrome, both of which are autoimmune diseases. An autoantibody is an antibody that attacks tissues of the organism that produced it. (How's *that* for gratitude?)

Dr. Lapp had noticed that normal cells treated with the green tea polyphenol, EGCG, showed significantly less SS-B activity than normal cells *not* exposed to polyphenols.

Really? We could actually quantify green tea's role in stifling the activity of a protein directly involved in autoimmune diseases? Amazing!

My excitement drove me into the lab of Dr. Lapp's husband, biochemist and molecular biologist David Lapp. In a room filled with computers and screens, he showed me data that were not only convincing, but consistent: EGCG inhibited human SS-B gene expression *more than threefold.*

Rolling Up Our Sleeves

It was clear to all of us that EGCG has a powerful effect on this protein, but we did not know how or why.

Several collaborators and I immediately rolled up our sleeves to learn more. We designed a series of experiments using both normal human skin cells and human cells that secrete saliva. We added EGCG to the cells and watched in astonishment as the polyphenol decreased the activity of *several* autoantigens, including SS-B. We wasted no time in submitting a paper to the *Journal of Pharmacology and Experimental Therapeutics.*

Only weeks later (approximately a nanosecond in research time), our paper was accepted for publication. Our hypothesis, "that green tea polyphenols could serve as an important component in novel approaches to combat autoimmune disorders in humans" [1], was now well on its way to becoming accepted science.

The ultimate goal, of course, is the most important: putting science to work for the betterment of mankind. Stay with me as we progress along that path....

REFERENCES

[1] Hsu S, Dickinson D, Qin H, Lapp C, Lapp D, Borke J, Walsh DS, Bollag WB, Stoppler H, Yamamoto T, Osakai T and Schuster G. Inhibition of Autoantigen Expression by Epigallocatechin-3-Gallate (the Major Constituent of Green Tea) in Normal Human Cells (2005) *J. Pharmacol. Exp. Ther.* 2005 315: 805-811

Chapter VIII

THE ULTIMATE BOUNCER

SUPPRESS, SUPPRESS!

I suspected a link between green tea consumption and Sjogren's syndrome because EGCG, that powerhouse of polyphenols, is known to suppress inflammation. Inflammation results when the immune system mounts a defense to a real or perceived enemy. Since EGCG suppresses inflammation, it should affect the magnitude of an autoimmune response.

How? My theory was that it does so by suppressing autoantigens. Autoantigens are normal molecules with useful functions, but changes in their amount or location can trigger an immune response. Suppress autoantigens and you suppress the immune response—which, in the case of an autoimmune disease, remember, is a good thing. We love the immune system when it attacks a virus. We're not so fond of it when it attacks our salivary glands.

To test my theory, I studied cells in salivary glands and skin tissue, exposing some to green tea and leaving the others undisturbed.

I expected to see *some* results, but I have to say, I was shocked by the magnitude. Cells exposed to green tea showed RNA and protein levels indicating autoantigen levels were suppressed in normal cells, but not in tumor cells. Once again, green tea was packing its remarkable double punch of attacking diseased cells while leaving healthy ones undisturbed. Talk about the ultimate bouncer!

Mouse Tracks

Because green tea had greatly diminished the levels of autoantigens in healthy cells, the immune system now had considerably fewer targets to potentially attack. This means a much lower risk of developing an autoimmune disease.

At least theoretically.

But remember, at that point, I had simply studied the cells in a Petri dish. My next step was animal studies.

My colleagues and I studied mice genetically bred to spontaneously develop autoimmune reactions against the salivary glands, tear glands and pancreas. Their symptoms included reduced saliva and tears—the same symptoms you would find in humans with Sjogren's syndrome—and increased blood sugar—a telltale sign of type 1 diabetes in humans.

When the mice became diabetic around the age of 15 weeks, their health deteriorated quickly. Most died within about two months.

So how would they fare if we treated them with green tea extract?

That's just what we set out to discover. We bred a new generation of the genetically altered mice. When they were nine weeks old, we began feeding green tea extract daily to half of them, while the other half went without.

We tested the urine of each mouse every other day, weighed them at the same time and made a fresh green tea extract "drink" daily for the treated group. For each mouse whose urine tested positive for glucose (indicating type 1 diabetes), we waited three weeks before collecting more urine and tissue samples.

Eye-Popping Results

It did not take long for astonishing results to materialize. The green tea drink simply changed these mice's medical destiny. The mice given the green tea extract had, among other things:

- Significantly fewer autoantibodies in the blood. (Remember, autoantibodies are produced by a faulty immune system to attack one or more of the body's own proteins.)
- Less salivary gland damage.
- Dramatically fewer lymphocytes—white blood cells that gather at the site of inflammation to fend off foreign cells in the case of healthy

individuals but that, in the case of Sjogren's disease, destroy salivary gland cells.

Our research team published the results in a 2007 edition of the highly respected scientific journal, *Autoimmunity* (8-1).

As impressive as the results were, was our study enough to prove that green tea protects us from autoimmune diseases? My answer was a firm *no.* More studies were needed. And there is no time like the present, right?

Revisiting the Mice

Our research team used a new generation of the same genetically altered mice to tweak the study a bit. This time, rather than feeding green tea extract to half of the mice at age nine weeks, we fed them EGCG (the powerhouse polyphenol in green tea) at age four weeks. Again, we left half of the mice untreated as a comparison group.

We periodically analyzed urine and tissue samples, supplementing traditional methods with exciting cutting-edge tools such as proteomics and genomics. This computer-assisted imaging and data analysis made our studies exponentially faster and more precise.

Our research, published in *Life Sciences* in 2008 (8-2), yielded several findings, but perhaps the most exciting is that EGCG consumption delayed and prevented type 1 diabetes in the mice.

Going Out On a Limb

Scientists always say that the more answers you uncover, the more questions you have. Type 1 diabetes is a complex condition, and I do not claim to have a magic bullet. But our findings have certainly whetted my appetite for further studies, and the importance of green tea cannot be ignored. In fact, I am prepared at this point to do something that researchers are generally loath to do—go out on a limb and make an unqualified declaration:

I think EGCG can delay and prevent type 1 diabetes in humans.

This admittedly bold statement is based not only on my team's studies, but on the fact that the disease is much more prevalent in the West than the East. We have already established that green tea is a mainstay of the Eastern diet, including during pregnancy and breastfeeding, so the average Asian is exposed to EGCG virtually from conception until death.

Yes, there are genetic differences between Americans and Asians, but can those differences alone account for the fact that the West has about thirty cases of type 1 diabetes for every two cases of the disease in Japan? That's a fifteen fold difference! Remember how many Japanese people consume green tea? Ninety-eight percent!

Dead Wrong

Another finding affected not just our understanding of green tea, but our understanding of autoimmune disease in general.

Before offering the details, let me share a bit of trivia: people with autoimmune diseases tend to have higher cancer risks than the general population. For instance, people with Sjogren's syndrome are at much higher risk of lymphoma, and type 1 diabetes increases the risk of pancreatic cancer.

Our research helped explain why. In studying the mice that, remember, were genetically bred to have symptoms including diminished saliva production, we found that the autoimmune reaction actually triggered the cells in the salivary glands to *grow*.

But these mice, like people with Sjogren's disease, didn't salivate *enough*. This fact has led to the conventional scientific wisdom that people with Sjogren's syndrome have *fewer* salivary gland cells, not more. After all, wouldn't *more* salivary glands equal *more* salivation?

No! We found that the conventional wisdom was not just wrong, but *dead* wrong (no cell related pun intended). We found in the mice that the autoimmune reaction did not *kill* the cells. It prompted them to proliferate … but with a twist. The mice's salivary cells grew in abundance, but they did not do what they were supposed to do: namely, salivate.

All of the mice, fed with water only, had salivary gland cells that did not seem to know what their function was. They were alive and well, but essentially useless.

We found that the cells were unable to receive a vital message to the brain: *to make saliva.* Our findings suggested that autoimmune diseases cause some kind of signal change that asks the cells to grow rather than work. The confused cells then put all their energy into proliferating, rather than carrying out their intended function.

Voila!

We then studied salivary gland cells of people who suffer from dry mouth (including those with the most common cause of dry mouth, Sjogren's syndrome), so we could compare mice to people.

Voila! The markers in their salivary glands indicated that, like the mice, they had too *many* cells undergoing proliferation, not too *few*.

At this time, another group published results that confirmed our finding: the salivary glands of healthy individuals do not receive a Go Forth and Hyper Multiply signal, but the glands of Sjogren's patients *do* (8-3).

Dry mouth, suffered by Sjogren's patients, is miserable in its own right (remember, dry mouth afflicts some 50 million Americans and can cause acute pain and/or discomfort), but the implications of this finding go far beyond this single disease. Remember the bit of trivia I shared earlier about autoimmune disease increasing the risk of cancer? Well, cancer is simply abnormal cell proliferation. Cells reproduce more than they are supposed to and form a tumor. And now we find that certain autoimmune diseases are characterized by abnormal cell growth? Of *course* there's a link! The same disease process is unfolding!

Common Denominator

It has long been known that another autoimmune disease, psoriasis, is characterized by abnormal skin cell proliferation. If we can find the common denominator in *all* of these disease processes—the source of the signal that tells cells to stop working and start growing—the potential for better health seems limitless.

And while we seek that elusive trigger, we are already finding wellness in a cup. A case study by the prestigious Mayo Clinic published in 2006 in the journal, *Leukemia Research,* showed that lymphoma patients showed significant improvement after taking a green tea supplement (8-4).

Based on this finding, the researchers gave varying doses of a green tea extract to patients in the early stages of lymphoma. Not only did the patients lack any adverse effects from even the highest doses of the extract, but most showed at least a fifty percent decline in lymph node size (8-5).

If green tea suppresses the growth signals for those nasty lymphoma cells, it no doubt suppresses signals for salivary gland cells. (See Chapter Three for more information about green tea and cancer.) My excitement is simply boundless.

The Sky's the Limit

There is still much more to know. For instance, I suspect that EGCG can turn on the body's defense system against TNF-α, a group of proteins and molecules involved in inflammation. TNF- α, which is produced by white blood cells, can reach out to target and kill cells—again, a *good* thing if the cells are diseased, but a *bad* thing if they aren't. In our results, salivary gland cells treated with EGCG had significantly fewer signs of cell death caused by TNF- α.

Obviously, much more work is needed—studies in Petri dishes, studies on lab animals and, if all goes well, eventual studies on humans.

But, oh, the possibilities! If green tea can help us battle those most mysterious and treatment resistant of maladies—autoimmune diseases—well, the sky's the limit.

Chapter IX

New Hope on the Horizon for Dry Mouth

A Horrible Affliction

I spent a considerable amount of time in Chapters Seven and Eight discussing dry mouth, or xerostomia.

If this problem—the inability to form sufficient saliva—strikes you as a mild inconvenience, or perhaps vaguely unfortunate, I guarantee that you have been fortunate enough not to experience it.

Dry mouth is a horrible affliction—and a huge source of suffering in the United States. Let us take a quick look at some of the particulars of a particularly loathsome condition:

- One of the main causes of dry mouth is Sjogren's syndrome, the autoimmune disease I extensively referenced in Chapters Seven and Eight. This syndrome affects up to four million Americans, most of whom are in the prime of their lives and about ninety percent of whom are women.
- Another common cause of dry mouth is medication. More than four hundred prescription medications cause dry mouth, regardless of age.
- Cancer treatment is becoming an increasingly common cause of dry mouth, as both chemotherapy and radiation can trigger the condition. More than 1.4 million people are diagnosed with cancer annually in the United States, so this side effect takes a considerable toll on quality of life.

- Dry mouth is also a potential side effect of diabetes, due to uncontrolled blood glucose. According for the U.S. Centers for Disease Control and Prevention, 23.6 million people in the country have diabetes.
- And perhaps the most regrettable risk factor for dry mouth is the one none of us can avoid, if we are lucky: aging. As I noted, dry mouth certainly is not an inevitable consequence of aging (note the low rate of the disease in Asia), but that is cold comfort for the people who suffer from it. About 30 percent of Americans age 65 or older (about 30 percent of that population) have some degree of dry mouth. If this condition continues to defy prevention or a cure, that number will skyrocket as baby boomers age. By 2030, a projected 71.5 million Americans will be 65 or older, and 30-40 percent of them will suffer from dry mouth.

All told, a conservative estimate of dry mouth sufferers in the United States is a whopping fifty million, and it is growing fast.

Cold Comfort

Currently, the only treatment for dry mouth is artificial saliva to lubricate the oral cavity, or stimulants, some of which are associated with side effects, to relieve the symptoms.

A prescription drug currently on the market for dry mouth has potential side effects including headache, visual disturbance, uncontrollable crying, sweating, respiratory distress, gastrointestinal spasm, nausea, vomiting, diarrhea, hypertension, shock, mental confusion, tremors and several heart related disorders.

The sad fact is that dry mouth can be so unbearable that these potential side effects are considered a fair trade off for even a modest measure of relief.

Can we design a new, better medication with all natural ingredients for dry mouth patients? I believe we can, with some key components, including, of course, green tea polyphenols.

HELP IS ON THE WAY

In early 2009, my employer, the Medical College of Georgia, helped me file a patent for a formula specifically designed for dry mouth patients, which is based on our previous patent for autoimmune diseases.

Unlike all other dry mouth products, this formula uses green tea polyphenols to suppress cell proliferation, inflammation and oxidative stress—the triple threat that lies at the very heart of dry mouth. (My students presented our research—including the finding that EGCG significantly increases antioxidant enzyme levels in animals—at the annual meeting of the American Association for Dental Research in March 2010.)

The next step? A study on humans to prove the formula's success in treating dry mouth. Thank heaven for my dream team of clinician colleagues, including oral medicine specialist Scott DeRossi, oral pathologist Kalu Ogbureke, salivary expert Douglas Dickinson and statistician Stephen Looney. I am playing merely a supporting role in the clinical leg of this research, but I am cheering on my colleagues every step of the way, confident we are on the brink of groundbreaking new treatment not only for dry mouth, but for other autoimmune diseases as well.

Stay tuned, won't you?

Chapter X

GOING VIRAL

A LOT TO SWALLOW

The information presented in this book thus far is, admittedly, a lot to swallow.

Can the leaves from a simple plant that grows in abundance really help treat cancer, obesity, skin conditions and autoimmune diseases, among other conditions?

As hard as it is to believe, I hope that the stringently researched evidence I have presented has helped you reach the same conclusion that I have reached: Yes, it can.

So will you hang in there while I make yet another seemingly amazing claim?

Green tea can kill viruses, too.

Am I kidding? Well, you be the judge, based on the information I will present shortly. But first, let's take a look at what *doesn't* work.

AN ALIEN INVASION?

No one loves China, my native land, more than I do, but a recent jarring experience illustrates the world's often misguided approach to infection control.

My wife, Tracy, and I took our two sons, Alex and Andrew, on a visit to China in May 2009. We wanted the boys, then ages six and seven, to know their roots.

But our welcome was less than cordial when our flight arrived in Pudong International Airport. Chinese border control officers boarded the Boeing 777 in supposedly virus proof gear that made them look more suited for a spaceship than a commercial plane.

Imagine my children's reactions when the officers pointed laser guns at our heads one by one to check our temperatures.

I thought fast to assuage my sons' fears. "Remember the movie, *Aliens?"* I told them. "The movie is showing in China, and the stars are here to reenact one of the scenes. Isn't this fun?"

Boy, did *that* do the trick. Not only did the boys' fears evaporate, but the border control officers suddenly became their best friends! Imagine the officers' confusion when the boys insisted on posing for pictures with them!

This is a great story in retrospect, but at the time, it was pretty unnerving . . . not only because my poor kids were initially scared half to death, but because it was so unnecessary.

Full Panic Mode

At that time, the world was in the throes of the initial H1NI, or swine flu, outbreak. The virus, which combines DNA strains previously specific to humans, birds and pigs, understandably caused worldwide alarm. The White House itself issued the solemn warning that half the U.S. population could be infected and as many as 90,000 (mostly children!) could die.

The Chinese government (as evidenced by our close encounter of the absurd kind on the plane) went even further, electing to quarantine fever plagued travelers. Chinese workers in South America were summoned back home. International plane travelers' body temperatures were checked upon arrival.

The government's intention was good—to create a flu free zone—but the policymakers were hopelessly naïve. Indeed, by late 2009, 80 percent of flu cases in China were H1N1.

Clearly, viruses have no respect for borders. Now that people, produce and animal products routinely zip from one part of the globe to another, the phrase 'it's a small world' takes on a whole new meaning. A global lifestyle ensures a global infection threat—if not from the virus de jour, then from the many that will inevitably follow in its wake.

The answer is not to panic or to enforce useless precautions. The answer is to be smarter than a virus.

Outsmarting a Virus

Our current infection fighting strategies are woefully inadequate. Vaccination, for instance, is useless if the virus has already entered the body or if the immune system is not fully functional. (This is why the very young and very old are at highest risk of death.)

How about using hand sanitizers to kill the virus before it can infect us? Yes, these products kill germs (99 percent, according to most of the manufacturers), but only for a few seconds. Yes, I said *seconds*. Let's say you apply hand sanitizer before leaving the house in the morning. Congratulations! Your hands are germ free until you reach for the doorknob in the bathroom where you applied the sanitizer.

Of course, viruses can also travel through the air . . . and trust me, they are smaller than the pores and gaps of any face mask you can find.

So if we cannot declare our bodies, our communities or our countries a virus free zone, what *can* we do? Aaahhh . . . this is where green tea comes back into the picture.

Nature's Way

On October 31, 2006, the U.S. Food and Drug Administration approved the first prescription drug containing active ingredients of green tea polyphenols to treat genital and perianal warts caused by the human papilloma virus. This is the first "drug" made of a botanical extract approved by FDA. More significantly, the extract is just a mixture of chemicals extracted by water from green tea leaves. It is completely natural.

Before being approved, this topical ointment was tested on hundreds of patients, both in the United States and Europe. The exciting results? The ointment cleared the warts in 53.6 percent of the study patients.

Great news . . . except for one thing: About twenty percent of the study patients reported side effects that included reddening of the skin, itching, burning, skin pain/ discomfort, skin ulcers, skin erosion, swelling, hard spots and rash with blisters.

A Potent Explanation

I can hear you crying foul this very moment.

"Hold it right there!" I imagine you exclaiming. "You've spent the last nine chapters telling us not only how great green tea is, but that it is virtually devoid of side effects, since our body simply excretes any excess green tea compounds through the urine."

Right you are. I have gone to great lengths to emphasize green tea's lack of side effects, not only because it is true but because it makes green tea products such potent weapons against illness and disease. So what's the deal with the wart ointment?

This ointment was made by very smart people; they put the water soluble green tea extract in an ointment preparation and specified that the ointment must be refrigerated before reaching patients. Why? Because the green tea extract is water soluble, quickly losing its potency when exposed to oxygen. Refrigeration does not halt oxidation completely, but it slows the process considerably—enough to produce the wart relief experienced by an impressive 53.6 percent of study patients.

To ensure enough extract will reach the wart, accounting for an inevitable degree of oxidation, the concentration of the extract is very high: fifteen percent. The high concentration also is necessary because the extract cannot efficiently penetrate the skin and cells (it is water soluble, remember) unless a high dose is loaded onto a very small area of skin. I believe the high concentration may account for the side effects.

This type of high dose is not natural, despite the natural ingredients in the ointment.

The question is: Can we lower the concentration to eliminate the side effects?

My answer is yes.

Coming Full Circle

In 2005, MCG filed a patent describing the use of lipid soluble green tea polyphenols for various uses in topical preparations, including anti microbial purposes. This group of green tea polyphenols is protected by a fatty acid group that prevents oxidation, and more importantly, optimizes skin penetration. Interestingly, when we tested the lipid soluble green tea polyphenols, we found that after entering the skin cells, they were converted to their original forms, such as EGCG [1].

In other words, capturing the healthful properties of green tea in a lipid soluble solution not only offers tremendous advantages (no worries about oxygen exposure, optimal skin penetration) but it does not detract one iota from the health benefits.

Have you come full circle with me at this point? The same green tea ointment that cleared genital and perianal warts in 53.6 percent of study patients—leading to an FDA approved prescription drug—can be captured in lipids, allowing a lower concentration that I think will significantly decrease or eliminate potential side effects.

Bound to Succeed

In 2002, an Italian research team reported in the journal, *AIDS,* that EGCG prevented the replication of human immunodeficiency virus (the virus that causes AIDS) in isolated lymphocytes [2]. However, this virus fighting ability required an extremely high concentration of the green tea polyphenol—a concentration too high to be sustained in the human bloodstream. Similar findings were replicated in subsequent studies [3], including a study determining that EGCG actually can bind to a protein called CD4 to prevent HIV from entering the cells [4] and that EGCG can prevent HIV from binding to the cells [5].

Yet another study at the University of Sheffield, UK used a very sophisticated method, nuclear magnetic resonance spectroscopy, to determine why: It seems that EGCG binds so tightly to the protein, there is no room for HIV to bind [6]. If the HIV cannot bind, it cannot infect.

In 2008, researchers in New York and Pennsylvania reported that EGCG can damage herpes simplex virus, the nasty bug that causes cold sores and genital lesions [7]. In fact, the same high concentration used in the Italian study inactivated the virus more than a thousand fold in just ten to twenty minutes!

How about the viruses that cause influenza, swine flu, bird flu and whatever flu? Well, as early as 1993, a Japanese group determined that EGCG can bind to a viral protein and inactivate influenza A and B [8]. Twelve years later, a more detailed study was reported from a group of Korean scientists. This time, H1N1 was included in the tests, plus two other strains [9]. At a quarter of the concentration used in the Italian study, half of the virus infection was inhibited.

ESTERS TO THE RESCUE

The conclusion: While we know EGCG can prevent HIV, herpes simplex and influenza infection, we still don't know how to apply it in humans, because drinking green tea may not be enough to kill the bugs. (Remember, our bloodstream will accept only so much EGCG, excreting the excess in urine.)

I think the answer might lie in handy little EGCG delivery systems called esters. Esters are compounds formed by a reaction between an acid and an alcohol, eliminating water. Esters are perfectly natural: These are the chemical reactions, for instance, that give wine much of its bouquet and aroma. Science has already shown that we can voluntarily initiate the process, for instance by packaging vitamin C in esters in dosages that otherwise would not be tolerated by the bloodstream.

In 2008, Japanese scientists at Osaka University published findings demonstrating that EGCG esters are 24 times more effective than the original form of EGCG in preventing influenza viral infection and inactivating the virus [10].

This is the proof I needed to validate the effectiveness of the patent MCG filed in 2005 for the topical use of lipid soluble green tea polyphenols.

Delivering polyphenols in lipid soluble compounds is not new, but the methodology has been virtually ignored since the first esters of green tea polyphenols were made in 1990s. (China and Japan obtained now- expired patents on the technology at the time.)

But the exciting promise of esters will not long be denied; their health enhancing potential is just too great. In addition to the applications I outlined earlier, I see other uses as well. For instance: remember the hand sanitizer I referenced earlier in the chapter? The product that keeps your hands beautifully germ free for all of maybe three seconds? I think esters are the solution to a longer lasting product. Laboratory tests have shown that hands coated with EGCG esters were protected against the H1N1 virus an hour after the esters were applied!

STAY TUNED

I am currently in discussions with a hand sanitizer manufacturer to propose adding EGCG esters to the product. A hand sanitizer that works longer than the time it takes to open a door? Hold on! It's coming.

I'm also interested in using EGCG esters for airway protection. Remember the limitations of a vaccine I outlined previously in this chapter? A vaccine cannot be developed until the virus is well under way, and therefore already wreaking havoc; it will not work in people already infected; and it will only help people with fully developed and noncompromised immune systems. Coating the airways with EGCGesters would preclude all these problems. Again . . . stay tuned.

So what exactly does all of this mean? I think it means that, very soon now, the healthful properties of green tea will be available in dosages and delivery systems that our body can tolerate with few or no side effects to fight not only the wide range of ailments I have already detailed, but to fight viruses as well.

Has any plant on earth ever proven as fruitful as tea leaves? And remember . . . we're just scratching the surface.

SIDEBAR

A Colleague and a Friend

The first EGCG ester was made by my good friend, Dr. Ping Chen, vice director of the Institute of Catalysts at Zhejiang University, China, where I serve as an honorary professor.

Dr. Chen passed his college entrance examinations at age fifteen and at a very young age became an associate professor and associate director of the Catalysts Institute in Zhejiang University, China's third ranking university. He is an expert in chemical reactions, knowing how to optimize conditions and select the most appropriate catalyst for a reaction between two or more molecules to form new molecules.

Dr. Chen was the first person to make EGCG at 99.999999 percent purity (100 percent, by scientific standards). Sigma-Aldrich, a leading chemical supplier, was Dr. Chen's customer because he was the only one who could supply such a highly purified EGCG. Today, Sigma-Aldrich sells EGCG in two grades-->95 percent and >80 percent--and they are very expensive . . . approximately $50 for 25 mg of the highest concentration, which is much more expensive than gold. (As of today, one ounce of gold costs about $1,000.)

Imaging the cost for EGCG at 99.999999 percent! Fortunately, we do not need such a high purity of green tea to receive the benefits. This comparison illustrates how hard it is to make something so pure. Dr. Chen is the person to meet that challenge. In addition, Dr. Chen was the first person to make EGCG esters. This work was published in 2002 and 2003 [11,12].

The improvement of methodology by Dr. Chen is a big step forward in green tea research, because we can test a purified single compound in laboratories and in animal models to understand the working mechanisms of the EGCG esters.

I was very impressed with Dr. Chen's work, so I went to visit him in Hangzhou, China several years ago. We chatted while enjoying Dragon Well (Lung Jing) green tea in China's most beautiful city. We have been good friends ever since; Dr. Chen sends me the best Lung Jing green tea each spring. In 2009, I had a chance to write a book chapter with Dr. Chen and my colleague, Dr. Douglas Dickinson, describing lipid soluble green tea in the *Handbook of Green Tea and Health Research,* published by this book's publisher, Nova Science Publishers Inc. [1].

How is that for coming full circle?

References

[1] Chen P, Dickinson D, and Hsu S. Lipid-soluble green tea polyphenols: potentials for health care and consumer products. Handbook of Green Tea and Health Research. Nova Publishers. 2009.

[2] Fassina G, Buffa A, Benelli R, Varnier OE, Noonan DM, Albini A. Polyphenolic antioxidant (-)-epigallocatechin-3-gallate from green tea as a candidate anti-HIV agent. *AIDS*. 2002 Apr 12;16(6):939-41.
[3] Yamaguchi K, Honda M, Ikigai H, Hara Y, Shimamura T. Inhibitory effects of (-)-epigallocatechin gallate on the life cycle of human immunodeficiency virus type 1 (HIV-1). *Antiviral Res*. 2002 Jan;53(1):19-34.
[4] Kawai K, Tsuno NH, Kitayama J, Okaji Y, Yazawa K, Asakage M, Hori N, Watanabe T, Takahashi K, Nagawa H. Epigallocatechin gallate, the main component of tea polyphenol, binds to CD4 and interferes with gp120 binding. *J Allergy Clin Immunol*. 2003 Nov;112(5):951-7.
[5] Hamza A, Zhan CG. How can (-)-epigallocatechin gallate from green tea prevent HIV-1 infection? Mechanistic insights from computational modeling and the implication for rational design of anti-HIV-1 entry inhibitors. *J Phys Chem B*. 2006 Feb 16;110(6):2910-7
[6] Williamson MP, McCormick TG, Nance CL, Shearer WT. Epigallocatechin gallate, the main polyphenol in green tea, binds to the T-cell receptor, CD4: Potential for HIV-1 therapy. *J Allergy Clin Immunol*. 2006 Dec;118(6):1369-74.
[7] Isaacs CE, Wen GY, Xu W, Jia JH, Rohan L, Corbo C, Di Maggio V, Jenkins EC Jr, Hillier S. Epigallocatechin gallate inactivates clinical isolates of herpes simplex virus. *Antimicrob Agents Chemother*. 2008 Mar;52(3):962-70.
[8] Nakayama M, Suzuki K, Toda M, Okubo S, Hara Y, Shimamura T. Inhibition of the infectivity of influenza virus by tea polyphenols. *Antiviral Res*. 1993 Aug;21(4):289-99.
[9] Song JM, Lee KH, Seong BL. Antiviral effect of catechins in green tea on influenza virus. *Antiviral Res*. 2005 Nov;68(2):66-74.
[10] Mori S, Miyake S, Kobe T, Nakaya T, Fuller SD, Kato N, Kaihatsu K. Enhanced anti-influenza A virus activity of (-)-epigallocatechin-3-O-gallate fatty acid monoester derivatives: effect of alkyl chain length. *Bioorg Med Chem Lett*. 2008 Jul 15;18(14):4249-52.
[11] Chen P, Wang H, Du Q, Ito Y. Purification of long-chain fatty acid ester of epigallocatechin-3-O-gallate by high-speed counter-current chromatography. *J Chromatogr A*. 2002 Dec 20;982(1):163-5.
[12] Chen P, Tan Y, Sun D, Zheng XM. A novel long-chain acyl-derivative of epigallocatechin-3-O-gallate prepared and purified from green tea polyphenols. *J Zhejiang Univ Sci*. 2003 Nov-Dec;4(6):714-8.

Chapter XI

GOING GLOBAL

TOO GOOD TO BE TRUE? HARDLY

As I have walked you through the health benefits of green tea in the preceding chapters of this book, I am mindful that skepticism may persist.

Maybe you are thinking: *This is all too good to be true.* Heaven knows we are inundated with enough spurious health claims to wonder if each new 'guaranteed product' is nothing more than snake oil.

But I am not selling a product. I am selling a message, and truthfully, a way of life. If everybody on earth began drinking three cups of green tea a day, I would be none the richer for it. But *you* would. I simply want to help spread the word that a natural, plentiful and inexpensive resource can dramatically improve your life.

Okay, so you are convinced I am not a snake oil salesman. But maybe you are thinking, "I'm healthy now. I don't need to drink green tea."

With all due respect, you cannot convince me that you are functioning at your optimal level of health. Americans spend more than two trillion dollars a year on health care, more than twice as much as the Japanese per capita and more than four times as much as the Singaporeans, yet our life expectancy is much shorter.

All countries with a longer life expectancy than ours—more than two dozen!—spend much less than we do on health care, no exception! And this is in spite of the fact that we have the best technology, medical research, innovation and health care training in the world.

Food for Thought

I know you have heard it before, but there is no escaping the fact that our diet and sedentary lifestyles are dooming us. Americans have the highest rate of obesity in the world, and with obesity comes heart problems, high blood pressure, diabetes and many other diseases. You need look no farther than supermarket shelves or fast food menus to realize that we are fueling our bodies with very poor quality calories. Even people who move here from other countries often see their health take a nosedive because of the American diet. A longitudinal study revealed that Japanese immigrants who maintain a Japanese diet after moving to the States have a lower risk for diabetes and heart disease than Japanese immigrants who adopt an American diet [1].

Frighteningly, the United States has begun exporting its poor quality diet overseas. Consider Okinawa, Japan, which once boasted the longest life expectancy in the world. Well, that good old time has passed. After American fast food invaded Okinawa, people got fatter and fatter. By the year 2000, the city had dropped from first to 26th in life expectancy among 47 Japanese prefectures [2].

Outlawing Obesity?

When I visited Japan, I saw fast food restaurants everywhere and limited access to fitness facilities. The country's obesity rate (still a relatively low seven percent, but quickly growing) has alarmed the government, which now spends fully a third of its health care costs fighting diseases related to obesity. In 2008, the government imposed drastic measures, actually "outlawing" obesity and mandating waist measurements. Men over 40 whose waistline exceeds 33.5 inches, and women whose waistlines exceed 34.5 inches, have six months to either trim down or receive nutritional guidance and "education."

And how are things going in Singapore? I have a particular interest in the country, having lived there from 1996-98 as an ESPN sports anchor. As I noted earlier, Singapore has a higher life expectancy than the United States yet spends a fourth of what we do on health care. How is this possible?

A Sporting Idea

The Singaporean government not only builds residential complexes that its citizens purchase at cost, but it offers huge sports facilities in every residential area—a total of 22. Those facilities feature Olympic sized swimming pools and children's pools (Singapore is hot every day); indoor courts for basketball, badminton and volleyball; steam and sauna rooms—you name it. My wife and I went to the sports complex often when we lived there, paying the equivalent of 80 cents a day. Sports facilities are also abundant in the Singaporean workplace. At age 40 plus, I joined a basketball team at ESPN.

The country is full of Western style fast food, but I think the fitness focus helps counteract the effects. The country also offers excellent health care insurance. The ESPN Asia insurance I had in Singapore covered virtually everything, with no copayments at all. Luckily for ESPN, my wife and I lived such a healthy lifestyle in Singapore that the only health care we need was dermatology and dentistry. I never had a sick day at ESPN.

So we have checked the pulse of health care in Japan and Singapore. How about my home country (as well as green tea's home country) of China?

Fast Food Invasion

Western style fast food restaurants are growing fast in China. Since the first McDonald's opened in China on April 24, 1992, more than 1,000 have followed in its wake. In fact, China is now the fastest growing market for McDonald's worldwide. KFC restaurants are even more prevalent—2,000 and counting since the first KFC opened in Beijing in 1987.* Franchises such as Pizza Hut and Burger King are hot on their trail.

The result? A 2002 survey conducted by the Chinese government revealed that 60 million Chinese people became obese between 1992 and 2002! That is about five percent of the population! China is on track to outpace the United States in obesity by 2020 [3], with similar consequences sure to follow: skyrocketing health costs and tragic obesity related diseases.

---

* When KFC first opened in China, Chinese people were dazzled by what they perceived as an upscale, fancy American restaurant. Young couples even wed at KFC! I'm not kidding; I actually attended one of these weddings in 1989. What a successful marketing story!

I am saddened that the Chinese government has seemed slow to react to this crisis. The same has been true in my adopted country of America. The federal government recently passed health care reform legislation that will hopefully alleviate some of our problems, but it is hard to imagine a sorrier state of affairs that the one we have had in recent years.

An Ounce of Prevention

Consider the plight of an acquaintance of mine whose first ten *days* of leukemia treatment cost $84,000. A half million dollar bone marrow treatment looms in his future. He lacks health insurance, which probably explains why five years of chronic inflammation went untreated. By the time he had no choice but to seek help, his disease had advanced considerably.

This is sadly typical of a health system that is treatment focused rather than prevention focused. The price tag will be enormous (in this case, with taxpayers footing much of the bill) and the prognosis is iffy at best. We should be very proud that we have the best doctors and technology, but we have to face the reality that we are a very unhealthy population. The only winner in this tragedy is the pharmaceutical industry, which relies on illness to keep the profits rolling in. I am grateful for lifesaving drugs, but frankly, our focus must be on prevention—not pills.

Carrot and Stick Approach

The good news is that our country demonstrates incredible resolve when push comes to shove. Our nationwide smoking cessation campaign is a good example. Too many Americans unfortunately still smoke, but the health risks are highly publicized, and society has largely stigmatized the practice.

Similar obesity cessation initiatives (some borrowed from our Asian friends) could help turn the tide. Our government could adopt a carrot and stick approach, such as building more fitness facilities while imposing a sin tax on bad calorie foods.

Those who profit from illness and empty calories will need to get on board, too. Fully seven of our country's top ten franchises are fast food restaurants. I applaud the fast food industry's willingness to add healthy options to their menus. Let us keep the momentum going, and let us discipline ourselves to limit fast food and empty calories to occasional treats. We need to exercise more, too. An old Chinese saying is, "Walk a hundred steps after dinner and live to age 99. Drink a cup of green tea after dinner and doctors will go hungry."

Of course, I do not want our doctors to go hungry. They are the best in the world, and they deserve to make a good living. But I hope that health care reform will reward doctors for prevention and minimize incentives for costly treatment of lifestyle related diseases.

MAJOR REVAMPING IN ORDER

Similarly, the pharmaceutical and health insurance industries need major revamping. In 2008, the top fifty drug companies employed 1.5 million people and made a profit of $1.28 trillion. (Yes, *trillion.*) In 2007, the top thirteen health care insurers and managed care companies logged combined revenues of $2.27 trillion, with almost $120 billion in profits. Such astronomical profits clearly indicate skewed priorities in our society. We have to stop popping unnecessary pills and start taking more responsibility for our own health.

The pharmaceutical industry needs to change its focus from drugs to botanicals, such as green tea extract. The precedent has been set; as I noted in an earlier chapter, the Food and Drug Administration recently approved Veregen (an extract of green tea polyphenols) to treat genital warts. I think the "drug" will soon be approved to treat certain types of leukemia as well.

THEIR LOSS IS YOUR GAIN

The pharmaceutical industry will not embrace botanicals willingly. The current emphasis is on artificial single molecule drugs, which are easy to patent and therefore more profit prone. Drug companies cannot patent green tea, green tea extract or any botanical extract. Their loss, but your gain. Botanicals are also largely free of side effects, and a big part of the pharmaceutical business is marketing drugs to treat side effects caused by *other* drugs. Fewer side effects obviously mean fewer drugs, and therefore smaller profits. Again: their loss, your gain.

I emphasize that I am *not* against drugs. They can and do save lives, relieve suffering and enhance quality of life. But drugs should be the exception, not the rule, in an average lifestyle. *Prevention* should be our benchmark, and green tea is an unparalleled resource toward this goal.

What do I do personally to advance this goal? Well, obviously, and as I have previously noted, I consume a lot of green tea, either in the form of tea, mints or gum. I use topical green tea products, such as skin care products, and take botanical extracts each morning for a good dose of vitamins and antioxidants. When I need to take medications such as antihistamines or pain killers, I try to balance them with herbs and other natural products. (To this day, I remember my graduate school mentor recommending a daily teaspoon of sesame oil to treat an allergy. After a few days, the allergy was gone.)

Botanical extracts are tried and true; indeed, herbal medicine was the *only* choice for most of the history of mankind. For example, the Chinese relied on traditional Chinese medicine (herbal and acupuncture) for five thousand years before they started using Western medications. In India and the Middle East, herbs have been used for thousands of years. Even in the United States, echinacea was one of the most prescribed medicines to fight infection before the discovery of antibiotics.

Getting on Board

Today, according to the World Health Organization, about eighty percent of the world population still uses herbal medicine. But they are never prescribed in American hospitals because they are not in "the book": the Physicians' Desk Reference. Every aspect of our health care system—medications, diagnoses, treatments, procedures, etc., must be by "the book"—regulations and rules made by medical authorities and the Food and Drug Administration. Of course, strict regulation can be a very good thing—but not if natural resources are left out in the cold. Our society's litigious nature does not help; sesame oil, for instance, is not "by the book," so any physician who prescribes it is setting himself up for an unwinnable lawsuit.

But as I noted, the precedent has been set for changing the rules. Veregen is already in "the book" to treat genital warts. Maybe sesame oil will find its way in "the book" soon, too. I think public demand, common sense and unsustainable health care costs will soon overwhelm the pharmaceutical industry's resistance to natural, nontoxic remedies.

The National Institutes of Health's National Center for Complementary and Alternative Medicine specifically funds research involving medicinal uses of foods, beverages, plants and herbs. The center has poured tens of millions of dollars into green tea research (no pun intended). The results have been astonishing and will just keep growing as more green tea containing "drugs" make their way into the pipeline.

We need to change the mentality that health care means disease treatment. We have seen the expensive and often ineffective results of a system based on illness. We need a system based on wellness, and every segment of society must get on board.

After all . . . our health is at stake.

SIDEBAR

Snack Attack

As course director for nutrition at the Medical College of Georgia, I am very mindful of what my young sons eat at home and in school. I worry about a culture that continually tempts them with junk food. All they have to do is turn on the television to be bombarded with ads for sugar loaded beverages and candies, salt laden chips and playground themed fast food joints. People raised in this culture tend to lose the ability to distinguish a healthy diet from an unhealthy one. Marketing works—for the marketers. *You are* the one left holding the price tag for triple bypass surgery.

At my sons' school, parents take turns sending daily snacks to the students. I campaigned hard to insist on healthy snacks. It worked for a few days, but soon, cookies and candies were sneaking their way back into the kids' backpacks. When pressed, the parents admitted that the unhealthy stuff is cheaper, more convenient and more popular than the fruits and all natural juices I championed. I finally waved the white flag. Now, my sons bring their *own* snacks to school.

REFERENCES

[1] Huang B, Rodriguez BL, Burchfiel CM, Chyou PH, Curb JD, Yano K. Acculturation and prevalence of diabetes among Japanese-American men in Hawaii. Am J Epidemiol. 1996 Oct 1;144(7):674-81.

[2] Akiko Yamamoto. Japan's New Public Health Problem Is Getting Big. Washington Post. June 19, 2007
[3] Levine JA. Obesity in China: causes and solutions. Chin Med J (Engl). 2008 Jun 5;121(11):1043-50.

Chapter XII

PICKING YOUR PRODUCTS

EMBRACING A LIFESTYLE

First, I need to say that there is no miracle drug, or miracle drink, or miracle green tea. There are a lot of scientifically validated benefits of green tea, including those generated by some of the best medical centers in the United States, such as the Mayo Clinic and MD Anderson Cancer Center. We now even have a "green tea drug" – Veregen, approved by the Food and Drug Administration.

But research into the therapeutic uses of green tea and green tea compounds is in its infancy. There are simply too many unknowns at this point to use green tea to treat a particular disease.

The good news is that scientists and clinicians, backed by the National Institutes of Health, are working very hard to find exactly how green tea battles disease and how to best deliver their disease fighting properties.

But in the meantime, the general health benefits of consuming green tea are indisputable. China and Japan celebrate green tea with "tea ceremonies," and I like this reverent approach to one of nature's finest gifts. Embracing green tea is more than a dietary change; it is a lifestyle change associated with a calm environment, a relaxed mind, a quiet moment, a way to nurture mind, body and soul with the healthiest beverage on earth.

A visit to a Chinese tea shop can be a little overwhelming. Believe it or not, China offers more than 400 brands of green tea. Differences include origins, shapes, colors, aroma, tastes and, of course, price. Even the United

States now offers dozens of varieties, not to mention associated products such as the gum and mints I helped develop.

Here are a few tips for navigating your way through the wonderful world of green tea:

LOOSE TEA LEAVES

Loose tea leaves are for true connoisseurs. Amateurs are welcome, but you better equip yourself with some knowledge.

I personally enjoy several brands of loose tea leaves. My most frequent pick is West Lake Lung Jing (Dragon Well) green tea, which is harvested in early spring on China's Shifeng Mountain of Hangzhou. Other favorites include jasmine tea from China's Zhejiang Province, the "Iron Buddha" brand of Wulong (Woo Lung) tea from Fujian Province, the "Silver Needle" brand of white tea from Fujian Province and "Pu Er" tea from Yun Nan Province. I drink Japanese tea on Japanese airlines.

White tea is very expensive due to the extremely "picky" picking rules: only new budding leaves with "hairs" on them are picked. (The tea is named for the hairs' resemblance to silver needles.) White teas, which are micro fermented at room temperature, smell so good, they can clear your mind immediately. White tea should be brewed in hot but not boiling water. (Approximately 90 degrees centigrade is a good benchmark.) The taste is very mild and sweet. The polyphenol contents are similar to those in regular green tea, so save your money if health benefits are your only consideration.

The most expensive green tea is the Royal Lung Jing (Dragon Well) spring green tea, which features a single budding leaf and a single young leaf. There is only one source of the tea in the world: the eighteen trees of the Royal Tea Garden[1]. The price can easily exceed $20,000 per 50 grams, or $11,200 per ounce. That is about ten times more expensive than gold! I have not tried it because it is not much different from tea grown nearby, which is much more reasonably priced.

[1] The Royal Tea Garden originated when Emperor Qian Long (1711-1799) visited a village in Hangzhou and noticed its residents picking tea leaves from eighteen trees by the well (named the Dragon Well because of its stone-carved dragon). He joined them, at which point his associate rushed over to deliver the news that the emperor's mother was sick. Qian Long placed his tea leaves in his pocket, then hurried to her side. She perked up when he arrived, asking, "What's that refreshing smell?" He reached into his pocket to retrieve the now dried leaves and asked servants to brew them and serve the tea to his mother. She quickly recovered, prompting the emperor to confer royal status to the eighteen trees.

West Lake Lung Jing tea, my personal favorite, comes from Hangzhou's Shifeng Mountain. Locals use a special water source, the Tiger Dogged (Hu Pao) spring in Hangzhou, to make this tea[2]. The tea is brewed slowly in water heated to around 95 degrees centigrade, unleashing a beautiful aroma. You can see the tea leaves change shape and color in the cup, leading connoisseurs to "pan fry" fresh leaves at a precise temperature to keep the leaves long, flat and green. Lung Jing is traditionally consumed from glass cups to ensure the integrity of the leaves.

"Iron Buddha"[3] is a brand of Wulong tea made in Fujian Province. The best is from Anxi area. The tea granules are very heavy, inspiring the first half of the name. Iron Buddha tastes very much like strong black tea because half of its polyphenols are oxidized. (Black tea, the most popular choice in the United States, is fully oxidized.) The oxidation decreases its healing properties, but the drink it still very healthful.

Jasmine tea comes from unfermented tea leaves dried with fresh jasmine flowers, creating a uniquely pleasant aroma.

The Chinese Tea Association assigns one of ten classes to teas, grading them based on outer look (shape, color, cleanness) and their properties in the cup (color, aroma, taste, leaf appearance) Each of these characteristics can be described in detail; connoisseurs want to know exactly what they are buying.

And if you are not a connoisseur?

I recommend selecting loose tea leaves based on smell (open the tin or container and sniff for freshness); appearance (teas should be even in size and shape, smooth and free of debris and abnormal growth); aroma (all good teas will have a pleasant, sustained, refreshing scent); and color (leaves should be bright with a little yellow and a little green).

Cheaper tea comes from leaves harvested in the fall. The taste is stronger and more bitter, but the health properties are comparable to those of more expensive teas. My suggestion is to sample a few brands, learn their

---

2 Folklore claims that Buddhist monk Jing Kong visited Hangzhou in 819 AD during the Tang Dynasty. He liked the place and wanted to build a temple there, but it lacked a water source. He dreamed of any elderly man telling him that two tigers would lead him to water. The next morning, Jing Kong saw two tigers digging in the ground. Water surged out, forming an everlasting spring. If you visit Hangzhou, stop by the Tiger Dogged spring (Hu Pao Quan) and drink the West Lake Lung Jing tea made of the water. It's the best.

3 According to the folklore, a tea farmer named Wei Yin had a dream one night around 1720. He had worshipped Buddha with a bowl of tea every day for decades, and in his dream, he saw a tea tree with round, thick leaves on strong branches. The next morning, he went to the mountains in search of the tree. When he found it, he transported it to his garden, considering it a gift from Buddha. He named the tea Iron Buddha and gave seeds from the tree to nearby farmers, perpetuating its goodness and generating a centuries old folk story.

backgrounds and associated folklore (just for fun!), brew them properly, rely on the "second pour" for your taste test (many people don't even drink the first pour) and determine your own favorites. You'll dazzle your friends when you start a conversation about your green tea expertise. It is amazing how much knowledge is associated with tea culture.

Tea Bags

I have to admit that I am something of a green tea snob. I have a clear preference for loose leaves; I find it very unlikely that the best green tea ever finds its way into a bag. (Remember, I grew and processed green tea as a child and have visited several processing plants. Trust me on this one.)

Not only is the quality of tea in loose leaves preferable to tea in bags, but storage is problematic for the latter. Bags left in open air at room temperature eventually lose their healthful properties. They should be stored as dry as possible; moisture hastens oxidation.

Of course, tea bags are preferable to no tea at all, but I am talking to a connoisseur at this point . . . right? Just remember: You get what you pay for.

Bottled Green Tea Drinks

What a wonderful idea: green tea in bottle, green tea to go! No more brewing with hot water, no need to add anything, just open it and drink!

Several years ago, a company asked me to help launch its bottled green tea in New York City. I politely declined because I did not want to destroy my reputation by making a false claim on something I do not drink.

Well, I'll qualify that statement a bit: I don't drink bottled green tea unless 1) I am thirsty, 2) no other type of green tea is available, 3) no clean tap water is available, 4) my only choices are bottled green tea or bottled water, and the latter is more expensive, and 5) the bottled green tea has no sugar or chemical preservatives.

Can you guess how much bottled green tea I have consumed in my life?

Green tea polyphenols are active antioxidants that react with oxygen in water. Bottled green tea means oxidized green tea, which means useless green tea, health-wise. This is why Asians never use leftover brewed green tea. Use it or lose it. (The health properties, that is.)

Strictly for research purposes, I am looking at a bottle of green tea now. It is labeled "Green Tea with Citrus," claiming "natural" flavors yet zero percent juice. How exactly do you get natural citrus flavors if your product contains no citrus? Natural indeed.

The label also states that the product has "72 mg of flavonoids antioxidant per serving" and 42 grams of sugars (and from high-fructose corn syrup . . . ouch!). So what I am holding is a highly processed, artificially flavored, sugar, salt and calorie laden drink with approximately zero health benefits.

China has cracked down on this kind of product, insisting on a certain percentage of polyphenols before a beverage can be labeled "green tea." (The wannabes are labeled "tea flavored beverages.")

I wish our Food and Drug Administration would follow their lead.

Tablets and Pills

I am not averse to green tea products, as long as they retain the health benefits of the real thing. (Remember, I helped develop green tea gum and mints.) But buyer beware. Read the label and look for "polyphenols" and "catechins" per unit. Avoid products with the word "extract" on the label, which suggests an "anything goes" amount of the good stuff.

But remember, more is not better when dealing with polyphenols. Do not exceed one gram per day; the excess will simply be excreted in the urine. Aim for small doses throughout the day.

Make sure that green tea products are dry and produced by a reputable company with a good track record of safety.

And remember that green tea tablets and pills are not as good for the oral cavity as green tea, which lingers in the mouth and throat.

Green Tea Extracts

Green tea extracts are often found in capsules and small bottles. Look for capsules with about 140 mg of green tea polyphenols. At this dose, you would need to take four to five capsules a day to receive the health benefits of green tea. And, as is true of tablets and pills, the capsules do not linger in the mouth and throat, so they do not offer the oral cavity health benefits of green tea.

As a reminder to stick with reputable companies with proven track records, here is an example of an online label of a green tea extract:

"A Proprietary Formula. A Liquid Dietary Supplement

Green Tea Max combines the power of highly-concentrated green tea PLUS a wide range of organic antioxidants. It has a high ORAC value. (Oxegen radical Absorbance Capacity). *Green Tea Max* contains organically grown green tea made into a concentrate with Vitamin C (100% RDI) and other antioxidants. It is more versatile than comparable green tea supplements. Green tea is a powerful antioxidant with high biological activity. Green tea contains the antioxidant effects of polyphenols and catechins with the power of EGCG (epigallocatechin-3 gallate), with versatile and potent health benefits.
Mix a full dropper of *Green Tea max* concentrate in hot or cold water for a tasty, healthy beverage. Substitute the healthy benefits of green tea for your coffee and get the "perk" with Green Tea Max. Add to your water bottle for aerobic activities.

	Amount Per Serving	% Daily Value
Green Tea Leaf Extract (90% Polyphenols, 30% EGCG)	200 mg	
Vitamin C	0	100%
Proprietary Blend (Grape Seed Extract, Pinebark Extract, Curcumin, Ellagic Acid, Magic Fruit Extract (Lohan), Citrus Bioflavonoids, Resveratrol, Selected Oligomeric Proanthocyanidins, Stevia Extract, Licorice).	100 mg	

Other Ingredients: USP Purified water, glycerin, natural lemon flavor.
Directions
Take one full dropper (2ml) 56 drops approximately, one to three times daily in a beverage of your choice.
Disclaimer
These statements have not been evaluated by the FDA. These products are not intended to diagnose, treat, cure, or prevent any disease."

Supplement Facts
Serving Size: 2 mL
Servings per Container: 75

I did not get farther than the misspelled "oxygen" in the second sentence before tuning out. But if you read on, you'll see that 100 percent of the recommended daily allowance of vitamin C is zero per serving! Come again? This manufacturer is obviously not reputable.

It is so amusing to me to read labels on some of the bottled green tea concentrates. One claims that green tea has been consumed in India "for thousands of years"! Hmmmm: Someone needs a geography lesson.

Suffice it to say that the only health benefit many of these products offer is the daily laugh I get when I read the labels.

GUM AND MINTS

Shortly after my colleagues and I published our findings on oral cancer in 2002, I received a phone call from Gary Blumenthal of the Philadelphia based company, TeaGuard. He wondered how many Americans could benefit from green tea. My short answer, of course, was "all," but I elaborated with examples of my research data. I thought that was the end of the conversation.

But Gary was not finished. He asked me what alternatives were available for people who did not like the taste of green tea or the bother of brewing it. His interest was both professional and deeply personal; he lost a family member to oral cancer. We had firm common ground.

I was moved by his determination to introduce the health benefits of green tea to convenience minded Americans. I visited him, then he visited me in my lab, observing our stringent research protocols. We soon determined that we could capture the healthful properties of green tea in gum and mints.

We knew it would not be easy; it is difficult to transfer enough green tea material into a new product to keep the health promoting catechins active. But after two years of work, we had developed several prototypes and flavors with different formulations. With the help of New Jersey based CCA Industries and New York based Ford Gum, we finalized the product and marketed it as Mega-T Green Tea Chewing Gum. The formulation is a trade secret, but pick up a package and you'll notice that each piece is separated and sealed in a blister pack to prevent exposure to air and moisture. Also, each piece is coated to further safeguard against oxidation. Inside the coating is the secret formula that offers a nice dose of green tea compounds in a great flavored, sugar free gum.

Each piece delivers a catechin concentration equivalent to two cups of green tea.

Next came our Mega-T Mints, boasting the same benefits as the gum. (A quick aside: the spearmint and peppermint flavors are very popular, but they inexplicably make me sneeze!)

We are continually improving the products. I hope to add the ingredient, xylitol, to further increase the oral health care properties, and we are improving the duration of a piece of gum. We are aiming for gum that lasts an hour, with the minty taste and health benefits lasting with every bite.

I always travel with the gum and mints, knowing my green tea "fix" is always within reach. (My perennially fresh breath is a happy side effect.)

So, if you are on the go, go with my green tea chewing gum and mints.

Skin Care Products

I discussed in Chapter Four how my Sudden Change green tea skin care line was developed. Suffice it at this point to emphasize that the products are effective and inexpensive. We are expanding the line to add products such as facial peels and masks. Remember, the products contain polyphenols in a formula that keeps them active and permeable to the skin layers. When they penetrate *live* skin cells, they start working right away!

As enthusiastic as I am about the products I helped develop, I am equally *un*enthusiastic about the many pretenders and wannabes on the market. Again, buyer beware. It is trendy these days to affix the words "green tea" to a label, but remember the product is basically useless if its formula precludes oxidation. Even the terms "clinically proven" and "dermatologist recommended" are suspect. Unless an ingredient in a skin care product is still active and fat soluble when opened, it cannot improve your skin.

Also beware the terms "complex" and "extract," which seem to be popping up everywhere. The more "extracts" in a product, the more it will cost. Plus, the more "complex" the ingredients, the less we know about how those ingredients interact. The real McCoy (i.e., my products) resulted from years of rigorous lab and animal testing. If a product does not meet these standards, you are better off buying a jar of petroleum jelly.

Looking Ahead

Many of the wannabe products I have referenced—and the many more that will follow in their wake—will probably quickly disappear once consumers experience the disappointing results. The ones with staying power are the ones that live up to their claims and, of course, good ol' brewed green tea.

As exciting as it has been to develop over the counter products with health and esthetic benefits, the next frontier is targeted medicine to treat specific diseases. I anticipate several cancer fighting green tea drugs will hit the marketplace shortly. I also anticipate new green tea dietary products, particularly those that promote weight loss. As the nutrition course director at the Medical College of Georgia, I always tell my students that weight loss and weight management require lifestyle change on several levels: eating right, exercising and, of course, consuming green tea! A single pill or compound, no matter how effective, will never substitute for a commitment to a healthy lifestyle.

In the pipeline for me are skin care products that target specific disorders, such as psoriasis and dandruff. I make no secret of my dissatisfaction with the current offerings on the market, many of which use the carcinogen, coal tar, and/or skin-thinning steroids.

I am also helping develop green tea products that specifically target dry mouth. (Want to get a head start on technology? Green tea in a cup is a wonderful weapon in your dry mouth arsenal.)

Finally, I envision a product line that uses EGCG esters to protect against viruses. The first virus I want to inactivate with the EGCG ester is the flu virus. Swine flu, bird flu and seasonal flu viruses have very similar protein coats, and lab tests show they can be inactivated by EGCG ester. If we can coat a layer of EGCG ester on the skin and in the nose, the risk of flu infection should plummet. EGCG esters also show promise in preventing human herpes simplex virus infection.

The trend seems very clear: green tea, revered for thousands of years for its healing properties, may help us more than our ancestors ever could have imagined. Meanwhile, I still love to drink slowly a few cups of West Lake Lung Jing green tea each day.

INDEX

N

O

P

Q

R

S

T

U

V

W

X